REIKI

PLAIN & SIMPLE

REIKI

PLAIN & SIMPLE

PHILIP JONES

THE ONLY BOOK YOU'LL EVER NEED

HAMPTON ROADS

Cover design by Jim Warner
Interior design by Kathryn Sky-Peck

Hampton Roads Publishing Company, Inc.
Charlottesville, VA 22906
Distributed by Red Wheel/Weiser, LLC
www.redwheelweiser.com
Sign up for our newsletter and special offers by going to
www.redwheelweiser.com/newsletter/

DISCLAIMER

*The information in this book is not in any way a substitute for receiving conventional medicine
or consulting a physician. All the practices in this book are to be used as an addition to existing
treatments to assist the healing process, and should be fully explored in only conjunction with suitable
training. Neither the author nor the publisher assumes any liability at all for any damage caused
through the application or misapplication of procedures and statements contained in this book.*

ISBN: 978-1-57174-785-3

Library of Congress Control Number: 2017958231

Printed in the United States of America

IBI

10 9 8 7 6 5 4 3 2 1

I dedicate this book to spiritual truth, Reiki, Mikao Usui, and all Reiki students.

I dedicate this book to ... Dr. ... Mike, ...
and all ... students

Contents

Invocation

May this book be a light in dark times and a bridge across the river of ignorance that leads you to achieve self-realization through the lotus chakra of love.

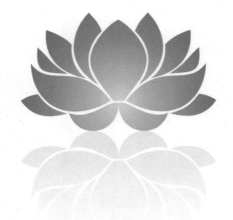

Acknowledgments

Thank you to my partner, Cerlin, and son, Jacob, for all their help and support, love, faith, guidance, and patience, and to my parents and family for their hard work, love, and tolerance and support.

I wish to thank all my family and friends who have supported me and my spiritual and healing work over the years. Without your contributions, this book would not have been written.

Special thanks to Simon and also to Sarah Blair and family for all their love and kind support.

Thanks to Chris for being a stepping-stone to the creation of this book.

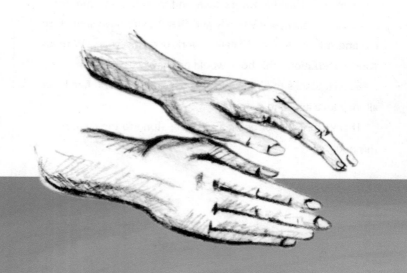

What
Is Reiki?

Reiki is a Japanese spiritual system used for self-healing, for healing other people, and for spiritual development. Two processes combine to make it work. The first is receiving Reiki initiations, which open your energy channels and connect you to spiritual energy. The second is using simple methods involving your hands, your eyes, and your intention to channel energy to a sick person or to use for your own spiritual cultivation. Students of Reiki should take particular steps to prepare for this work. There are also specific methods within Reiki that differ from faith healing or spiritual healing as understood by healers, channelers, and mediums around the world.

This book will not take the place of initiation. There is certain information that can be acquired only through initiation, and that information will not be contained here. What this book will give you is a good introduction to the healing power of Reiki, and it will help you channel your healing intention.

The word "intention" often crops up in books about healing these days and is clearly developing a new meaning, not familiar to the world in general. Intention in this context doesn't mean that one is *planning* to do something; instead, it signifies that one *intends* to do something good, worthwhile, and desirable.

Reiki students receive initiations from Reiki teachers so that they are awakened and connected to the universal energy. The connection process opens their energy channels to Reiki and links them all the way back to the founder of Reiki, Mikao Usui. This "energetic link" acts as protection as well as an unseen form of guidance for students while they are using and working with Reiki.

To heal with Reiki, the practitioner lays his or her palms on a sick person while allowing the energy to flow into the patient. Practitioners do not need to intervene with the channeling of the Reiki, as it automatically flows through them once their energy channels have been opened, and once they have the intention for healing. They simply place their hands in specific hand positions on a person and allow the energy to do its work. Practitioners do not have to visualize anything while using Reiki; they may simply stay in the present moment or focus their minds on the *hara* in their lower abdomen.

The *hara* is an energy area located three finger widths below the navel and about an inch inside the abdomen. Focusing on this area allows the mind to stay calm and helps to build great quantities of energy in the body during the treatment. As practitioners progress, they move away from the systematic hand positions (which are shown later in this book), because the Reiki guides healers so that they use their hands as energy sensors. This system enables practitioners to feel energy imbalances in a sick person. It also allows the consciousness of Reiki to move practitioners' hands anywhere on and around the sick person, without the healers' judgmental minds and egos getting in the way. This method is taught to all new first-level Reiki students; however, it takes time, practice, and confidence to master. This ability is awakened through Reiki empowerment.

Reiki is much more than just a healing system; it is also used to develop spiritual awareness, which will help you to live a happy life. This was the fundamental teaching of Mikao Usui. Regular spiritual empowerments, the twenty-one-day palm-healing cleanse, meditations, breathing exercises, visualizations, mantras, mystical symbols, and five Reiki precepts are the aspects of Reiki that make it unique as a healing and spiritual system.

The word "Reiki" is made up of two Japanese kanji characters (*kanji* is an ancient Japanese writing system). The first character, *rei*, means "spiritual" or "soul." The second character, *ki*, means "energy," which consists of the vital forces of the Earth and universe. Therefore, the Japanese meaning of the word "Reiki" is "spiritual or soul energy." However, in the West, the word "Reiki" is generally understood to mean "universal life force energy." This was thanks to Hawayo Takata, a Reiki teacher who introduced Reiki to the West. She believed that Reiki contained universal energy, or life force energy.

To this day, very little is known about the nature and origins of this spiritual energy. What we do know is that it was brought into the wider world via the hard work, focus, and open heart of Mikao Usui. Thus, all types of traditional and nontraditional Reiki must ultimately lead back to the founder, Mikao Usui. Usui was a Buddhist who lived at a time when Buddhism and Shintoism were practiced side by side. He also practiced and studied many different mystical arts, as well as martial arts and a system for cultivating and mastering energy, called *"kiko."*

Usui is said to have studied Buddhist sutras (discourses by Buddha), which led him to his spiritual experiences and the awakening of Reiki. We know also that some of the symbols and mantras in the system of Reiki are Japanese Buddhist and Shinto in origin. Some are also in Sanskrit, an ancient Indian language, more than two thousand years old. We can therefore say that

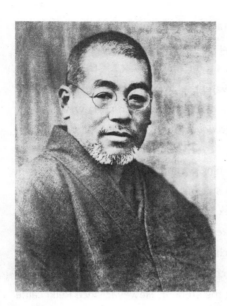

Reiki master Mikao Usui,
(1865–1926)

beyond Usui, the Reiki, or spiritual energy, extends back as far as Buddha, Shinto gods, early Indian mystics, and the very source of light itself. I am talking not of the system of Reiki itself, but of the stream of energy represented by the word "Reiki."

We can use Reiki methods to access, cultivate, and utilize spiritual energy, to allow every human being to discover his or her true self, regardless of culture, color, creed, or religion. This is known as self-realization, and it is the first moment of discovery, when one understands who one truly is. This self-realization or enlightenment gradually grows in a person, and the light is reflected through that person's heart, to be shared with the world. This is about not just peace, but cutting the cord of ignorance so that spiritual truth and love can be felt in their pure, formless essence.

Mikao Usui was a catalyst for the light to allow the world to have a channel and an anchor for that light, so that it could be accessed by mere touch, a thought, or a look. He taught methods that brought spiritual awareness, truth, knowledge, healing, and love for all beings. These methods would create a wave of light over the world, helping to develop the spiritual evolution of each soul upon the earth.

Usui's method of teaching was open-ended, so that each person received training to suit his or her requirements and capabilities. There was no specific time limit for each level; when Usui thought students were ready to move on to the next level, he initiated them into it. Achieving proficiency in the methods and energy at various levels could take from a few months to five or ten years, depending on the student. However, once Reiki came to the West, a system evolved to ensure that students had at least three to six months of experience in one level before moving on to the next. This system creates a good foundation. Sadly, this is not the case with all Reiki training in the West today, as some first- and second-level Reiki courses are taught together over a weekend. In my view, this makes it difficult for the student to digest the energy and teachings in a pure and simple way. There is no space and time for growth, cultivation, and experience with the different energies and methods. I feel that a Reiki student can gain a great deal of personal, spiritual experience with a little time and patience. Patience is one of the fundamental qualities that need to be developed by all teachers and students who follow a spiritual path.

It is interesting to note that, in earlier times, the system of Reiki was given many different names. Usui didn't actually give it a name himself, but according to the inscription on his tombstone, he did refer to it as "Reiho," which means "spiritual methods."

The spiritual methods in this book have been specifically chosen to help you on your path of love, light, healing, and self-knowledge.

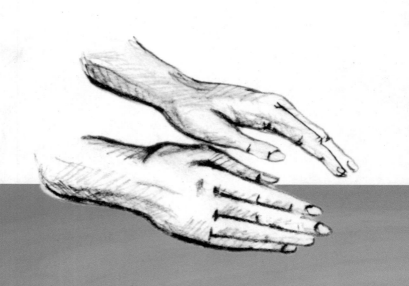

Origins
of Reiki

1

What makes Reiki unique? This question is asked by many people in the alternative healing field of work.

The first and most obvious answer to this question is that Reiki was founded and introduced to the world by Mikao Usui, a Japanese Buddhist lay monk who was a master of martial arts, energy cultivation, and many other mystical Buddhist and Shinto practices and healing methods. It was a culmination of his efforts, knowledge, compassion, and grace that helped this system to develop. All systems of Reiki should therefore be traced back to Reiki's origins in Japan and to Mikao Usui. This is called the "Reiki lineage," and all students, whether they are aware of it or not, are part of a lineage of teachers and students that extends all the way back in time to Mikao Usui.

The Reiki lineage goes deeper than simple historical links, as it has an "energetic connection" (i.e., a connection to the spiritual energy called Reiki). It is this energetic connection and the initiation between the teacher and the student that make Reiki different from other healing systems.

Reiki Lineage

Mikao Usui

Mikao Usui was born on August 15, 1865, in a village that was once called Tania Mura (now called Miyama-Cho) in the Yamagata district of Gifu in the former Japanese capital of Kyoto.

His father's name was Taneuji, but he was commonly called Uzaemon. His mother was from the Kawai family. They had a daughter and two more sons, and were a Tendai Buddhist family. Usui married Suzuki Sadako, and they had two children, a girl named Fuji and a boy named Toshiko. Mikao Usui was a large and sturdy fellow, stouthearted, gentle, modest, and tolerant. He had a practical nature and he took great care with his tasks.

Usui was introduced to martial arts and *kiko* (energy cultivation) at a young age when he entered a Tendai Buddhist monastery near Mount Kurama. From the age of twelve, he studied and trained in a particular martial art called *yagyu ryu*, which is a system of samurai swordsmanship. He became very proficient at this art and, in his twenties, attained the level known as *menkyo kaiden*. Usui trained in many other ancient Japanese arts, in which he also reached a high level of proficiency, and he became well known and respected by many other high-level martial arts practitioners and masters of the time.

Beginning in 1922, Usui trained in Zen Buddhism for three years. It was also in 1922 that Usui established his first healing group and center in Harajuku, where he offered training and healing in Reiki *ryoho*, the Reiki spiritual method. This center was called the Reiki Ryoho Gakkai. In 1923, in Japan, a large earthquake killed or injured many people. Mikao Usui went out daily during this period to treat and help the injured with his methods. He is said to have saved many lives during this period of disaster.

As an older man, he visited Europe and America, and he studied in China. By nature, he was versatile and creative, and he loved reading many different kinds of books. He studied history and medicine, Buddhist and Christian scriptures, and psychology, Taoism, divination, incantation, and physiognomy. All Usui's

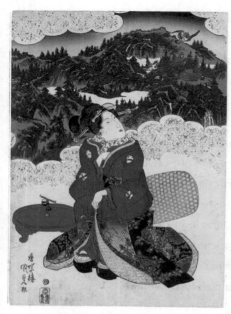

Mount Kurama, from the book *Inaka Genji* by Tanehiko (Museum of Fine Arts, Boston)

experience and knowledge of life surely must have influenced him and encouraged him to discover his spiritual path and the Reiki system.

Hiroshi Doi, who was once a member of the Usui Reiki Ryoho Gakkai, and who is an influential figurehead in the Reiki world today, says that Mikao Usui sought the ultimate purpose of life, to be enlightened and to implement that enlightenment in the world for humanity. To this end, Usui went to Mount Kurama in Kyoto, where he fasted and meditated for twenty-one days; on the twenty-first day, he suddenly felt a great Reiki over his head, and at this point, he finally achieved enlightenment.

As Usui's fame grew, he was invited to speak at many venues, where he demonstrated what he had learned. Eventually, he reached the city of Fukuyama, where he suffered a stroke. He died very unexpectedly on March 9, 1926.

Dr. Chujiro Hayashi

Dr. Chujiro Hayashi, born in 1878, was a forty-seven-year-old retired naval officer and doctor when he spent a year training with Mikao Usui. He had been a member of the Usui Reiki Ryoho Gakkai, but in 1932 Dr. Hayashi set up his own clinic and society.

Dr. Hayashi noted down details of all the treatments and methods in the Reiki system in a healing guide, which he called *Ryôhô Shishin*. It was through Dr. Hayashi's research and medical background that the twelve basic hand positions were established. Even with the healing guide, Hayashi expected his students to be proficient in advanced scanning (using the help of Reiki spiritual guidance to sense what ails the client) and intuitive healing methods.

Japan was about to enter the Second World War, and as a former naval officer, Dr. Hayashi was expected to support the war effort. He didn't want to be involved in war, however, so, sadly, on May 10, 1940, Dr. Hayashi took his own life.

Hawayo Takata

Hawayo Takata, a Japanese-American widow with two children, was born in Hawaii in 1900 but lived in Japan. Takata first came into contact with Reiki in 1933, when she was suffering with depression and a tumor, along with many other ailments. Her doctor told her that she would have to undergo surgery to remove the tumor. While Takata was in the operating theater awaiting her operation, her dead husband spoke to her repeatedly, saying, "The operation is not necessary. The operation is not necessary." She aborted the surgery, and then asked her doctor if he could recommend someone who used traditional healing methods. One of the doctor's family members had been successfully treated at Dr. Hayashi's clinic, so the doctor referred Takata there.

Takata went to Dr. Hayashi's clinic and received daily Reiki treatments from three Reiki healers for several months. Initially she was quite skeptical of the palm-healing method, but she became intrigued by the amount of heat her Reiki healers produced from their hands and the feeling of well-being this seemed to produce in her. After several months of Reiki treatment, Takata was well again. Naturally, her interest in Reiki and palm healing grew, and she wished to learn the practice for herself. She moved in with Dr. Hayashi and his family and trained in the system for more than a year. Takata then returned to Hawaii, where she practiced and gave Reiki treatments. Sensing that war between the United States and Japan was inevitable, Takata returned to Japan, and in 1938 Dr. Hayashi initiated her as a Reiki master. She eventually returned to Hawaii and set up a Reiki clinic there, training a further twenty-two people as Reiki master teachers before she died on December 12, 1980.

Takata's granddaughter, Phyllis Lei Furumoto, and Dr. Barbara Weber Ray carried on the Usui Shiki Ryoho system of Reiki. Eventually, Furumoto was elected Takata's successor as head of the Usui system of Reiki.

What Makes Reiki Unique?

The following methods make Reiki unique and distinguish it from other forms of healing.

Reiki Initiations

Reiki initiations are called "attunements" in the West and *"reiju"* in Japan. Unless they receive these ancient attunement processes from a Reiki master, students are not practicing Reiki. Mikao Usui gave regular *reiju* empowerments, or attunements, to his students. These attunements passed on the Reiki, and opened and empowered particular energy spots and channels within the students, enabling them to access Reiki whenever they wanted. It is these initiations that connect the student to Reiki and Usui for the rest of his or her life.

Reiki is accessible to everyone because it doesn't require students to be familiar with any other form of healing or energy work, nor is there any need for students to be particularly spiritual or religious. Students may believe in spiritual energy or they may not, but either way, the attunement/*reiju* process will be activated and will do what it is supposed to do. Reiki is nonjudgmental and has a compassionate quality that allows it to accept all beings regardless of their beliefs, experience, faith, race, or status. The attunement/*reiju* process has been passed down through the years, beginning with the founder, Usui, and continues to the present day. It is this process that allows each person to open up to and be empowered by Reiki.

Twenty-One-Day Palm-Healing Cleanse

Another aspect that makes Reiki different from other healing systems is the twenty-one-day palm-healing cleanse. This healing cleanse ensures that you experience Reiki over a period longer than the two days in which you receive your training. For an hour each day over twenty-one days, you give yourself a Reiki treatment using twelve basic hand-healing positions. This gives the Reiki a chance to really open your inner energy channels and work through your body, emotions, and mind. This process removes inner energy blockages that may be encountered as reactions in the mind, emotions, or body, and it brings balance and harmony.

This will make you happier and more peaceful, and it gives you a firm foundation for giving healing to others.

Reiki Symbols and Meditation

The mystical Reiki symbols are sacred and will not be revealed in this book. The symbols are introduced into the Reiki system at the second level. I consider the use of the symbols as the science of Reiki. There are four original Japanese Reiki symbols. Two of them are in ancient Sanskrit, and the other two symbols are kanji characters. They allow the student to access particular spiritual states of consciousness and energetic qualities. Usui introduced the symbols into the Reiki system for those students who found it difficult to chant and meditate using the *kotodama* (word spirit) mantras. These symbols can also be used to bring the same qualities and energies into a patient during healing.

Within the system of Reiki there are many different meditations, and some of these will enable you to generate more Reiki in your body and soul, making the soul more powerful, the body stronger, the mind more peaceful, and the emotions more balanced. There are also meditations to develop and become one with the different qualities of energy and the higher spiritual states. These methods originated from Buddhism, Shintoism, and *kiko*, which is the Japanese practice of mastering and cultivating energy.

Reiki Mantras and Kotodama

The Reiki mantras are introduced at the second level also. The mantras are ancient words that are chanted a number of times to invoke divine vibrations in the body and in the spiritual heart and consciousness. These mantras provide swift access to the power of the Reiki symbols.

The *kotodama* are very old mantras that can be chanted independently of the Reiki symbols, yet can be used to access the same power of the symbols. Again, the mantras and *kotodama* can be mentally chanted during healing to invoke their energetic qualities in your patient.

To learn the mantras and symbols correctly, you need to study with a Reiki teacher in a second-level Reiki workshop, sometime after completing the first level.

It is all these elements of the Mikao Usui Reiki system that make Reiki unique compared to other healing and spiritual systems.

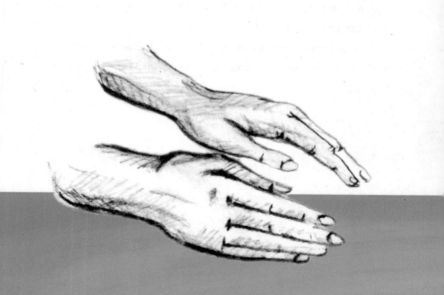

The Five
Reiki
Precepts

2

The five Reiki precepts are really the foundation of the Usui Reiki system. These precepts enable you to live a happy, healthy, peaceful, and spiritual life. Even if you didn't practice any of the other methods incorporated in the Usui Reiki system, and practiced just the five precepts daily, you would make rapid progress on your spiritual path to truth. This shows just how powerful these precepts are.

The five precepts were called the *Gokai*, and they are written on Usui's tombstone like this:

招福の　秘法
萬病の　靈薬

今日丈けは　怒るな

心配すな　感謝して

業をはげめ　人に親切に

朝夕合掌して心に念じ
口に唱へよ

心身
改善　臼井靈氣療法

肇祖　臼井甕男

In English, the message looks like this:

> The secret method for inviting happiness through many blessings, the spiritual medicine for many illnesses.
>
> | Just for today: | Kyo dake wa: |
> |---|---|
> | Anger not | *Okoru na* |
> | Worry not | *Shinpai suna* |
> | Show gratitude | *Kansha shite* |
> | Work hard | *Gyo o hage me* |
> | Be kind to others | *Hito ni shinsetsu ni* |
>
> Mornings and evenings, sit in **gasshô**. To do this, you kneel and sit on your heels, and then you put your hands together as though you were praying. Repeat aloud, and recite in your heart: "For improvement of mind and body."
>
> **Usui Spiritual Healing Method**
> **The Founder: Mikao Usui**

There is speculation among Reiki practitioners about the origins of Usui's precepts. They may have been adapted from earlier Japanese religious texts that predate Usui. Usui placed great importance on the practice of these precepts, as they were considered to be a way of inviting happiness and blessings into one's life. According to Usui, they are the spiritual medicine for all illnesses, and they should be practiced daily to improve the mind and body.

Practicing the Reiki Precepts

You may practice the five Reiki precepts using the procedure outlined on Usui's tombstone:

1. Find a private place in your home, or use one that you regularly choose for meditation.

2. Kneel with your feet tucked under you, or sit cross-legged.

3. Mentally ask for the Reiki to come in, and then feel the flow of gentle energy.

4. Put your hands in the prayer position (*gasshô*) at your heart (shown on page 23).

5. Repeat the five precepts out loud, and feel in your heart and meditate on what you are saying. If it is difficult to repeat the precepts out loud, you may say them quietly or simply think them.

6. Perform this ritual for five minutes in the morning and evening.

Practicing this method will make you more aware of your thoughts and actions. You are consciously instilling a positive habit into your heart and into your subconscious. The practice will start to overflow into your daily life: you will worry less about unimportant matters, and you won't get angry and overreact to situations that seem to be beyond your control.

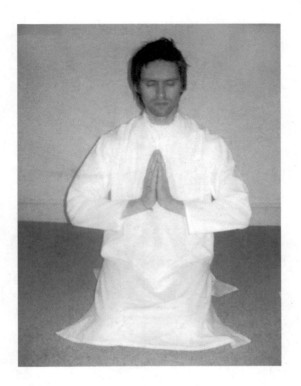

Note:

Be patient and kind to yourself when practicing this method because you may become aware of the extremes of your thoughts and emotions for a while.

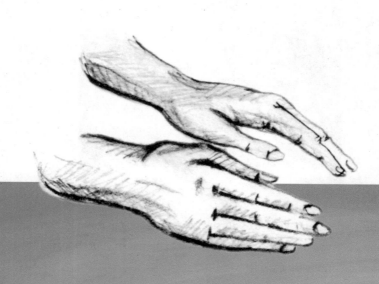

Finding
a Teacher

3

Finding a suitable Reiki teacher can take time. Sometimes a teacher seems right at first, but after a time you may feel the urge to move on to another. This is fine, as long as your knowledge and practice are deepening and you maintain a spiritual view and respect all those who give you information. Try not to become a spiritual junkie, chasing one spiritual experience after another, because you will only become confused and disillusioned. I've trained with three Reiki masters over the years, and each taught me something worthwhile, bringing a measure of spiritual insight and gifts into my life. Each master came along when most needed.

Finding the right teacher is a process of trial and error, so I recommend that you read up on the subject, look on the Internet, go to a couple of introductory lectures on Reiki, or have a treatment. Even a brief treatment at a demonstration event can be enough to whet your appetite. Most of all, listen to your heart. Ask yourself if a certain teacher feels right for you and if you are right for the teacher. Remember, having the title "Reiki master" doesn't ensure that the teacher is enlightened or more spiritual than you are. The only differences between a Reiki teacher and you are knowledge and practice. You may find that a teacher comes into your life just when you least expect it and without much effort on your part. Even so, don't assume that this teacher is perfect for you, but maintain a level of discernment and common sense, while keeping an open mind and an open heart.

Absolutely anybody can learn Reiki, regardless of religion, faith, or experience. All you truly need is the desire to study, practice, and receive the empowerments. Above all, be openhearted. Even if you don't believe in "subtle energy" or "esoteric knowledge," the fact that you are reading this book means that you are being affected by Reiki in some way, and your heart is opening to some degree, whether you realize it or not.

If you take your study of Reiki further, you will find that after just two days of Reiki training at the first level, your Reiki channels will be opened—and they will stay open for life. Your teacher will give you a set of personal tools that will enable you to give healing to yourself and to others in a systematic way. You will also discover meditations and breathing exercises that enable you to build up and store the Reiki, and principles that allow you to live a peaceful life.

A Reiki Course Group

Once you find a Reiki teacher that you trust, take the plunge. Newcomers start with the first degree, though some people teach the first and second degrees back to back over a weekend. The size of the group depends on the teacher and the facilities that are available. My personal training always took place in groups of five to eight people. However, when I reached the higher levels—the third degree and the teaching degree—the group usually dwindled down to one or two people. In Japan, large groups can fill a hall, with empowerments taking place for everybody simultaneously.

A group usually starts with a method called "Reiki *mawashi*" which means an "energy circle." This is a great way to start a course, as the Reiki energy passes around the circle through each person's hands. This process removes tension and anxiety, is very relaxing, and can be the start of a healing process for some students. Each student gives a brief outline as to how and why he or she decided to participate in a Reiki course. The groups are usually very relaxed, supportive, and informative. They are also very practical, as there is always time for questions and answers.

Initiation

The Reiki teacher uses an ancient Japanese initiation to open the Reiki student's energy points and channels. The Reiki initiations originated from ancient Buddhist empowerments, but you don't need to be a Buddhist to receive them. In the West, we talk of "Reiki attunements," but Japanese Reiki initiations are called *reiju*, which means "spiritual gift." Once you have received the Reiki initiation, you have a channel to Reiki for life.

I will not describe the actual attunement process in detail in this book, because it is taught only to students at the teacher level—those who think it is their life's path to teach after completing all the other Reiki levels. Reiki teachers around the world use a variety of subtle differences in method.

The more you practice Reiki, the more the Reiki channel opens and strengthens, so that your connection to the spiritual source becomes reinforced, allowing you to access a higher level and greater quantity of the spiritual energy. Even if you decide not to practice Reiki for many years after your initial training, you will still have access to the Reiki if you decide to use it again. Students who leave aside their Reiki for a long period suffer from self-doubt about their Reiki connection and their healing ability, but they soon realize that it hasn't gone and that the connection is still there. If this happens to you, I suggest that you treat yourself to a Reiki workshop or participate in a Reiki share group. In this way, you can practice your healing and meditation and receive a Reiki initiation again, just to reinforce your connection and belief in your channel to Reiki.

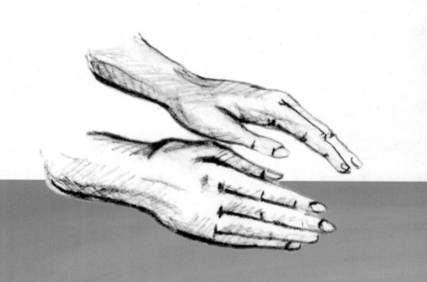

Attunements

4

The Western attunement process can be quite a long, drawn-out affair, so if you are last in your Reiki group to receive it, you may have to wait a while. You and all the other Reiki students sit in a circle on chairs, facing outward. A Reiki teacher will tell you beforehand what he or she is going to do and what you have to do, and then the teacher gives each student his or her first Reiki attunement individually.

You and the other students sit in a meditation posture called *gasshô*, holding your hands together in prayer around your heart area. The Reiki teacher will gently place his or her hands on certain areas around your head and upper body, while following a meditative procedure. Through this gentle process, the student is empowered with Reiki, and certain energy channels are opened.

The energy points and channels that are gently awakened are the crown and the central energy channel, which flows from the head to the base in the body. Other centers that are now opened are your spiritual (third) eye, your spiritual heart, and the channel running from your heart through your arms to your hands and palms. Whenever you give healing or meditate with Reiki, these subtle energy channels become stronger, allowing more Reiki to flow through them.

Some students experience phenomena such as light, heat, or cold during attunement. Some see colors, or feel tingling or aches in the body, heaviness or lightness of body, peace, euphoria, laughter, tears, and many other sensations. This is not the case for all students, however; some get very mild sensations, if any. These sensations and experiences do not mean that the attunement is good or bad; each student is starting a spiritual and energetic purification, and all will be awakened to Reiki, regardless of their personal experiences from the attunement. The Reiki teacher finishes the attunement by sealing the channel of Reiki. This can be done using visualization, intention, and Reiki symbols.

At this point, some teachers tell the students to rest their hands on their thighs with their palms facing downward to allow the flow of Reiki to circulate through them while the teacher gives attunements to the rest of the group. To finish the attunement, the Reiki teacher may then bow to the student or say, *"Namaste,"* which means, "I bow to the divine within."

The attunement process that I have just described may not be the same for all teachers; it is just an example to give you an idea of what you may expect during an attunement process. For example, I received four Reiki attunements over a two-day period for each of the Reiki levels during my training. I therefore give the same number of attunements to all of my students, in addition to distant attunements after the course has been completed, and further ones in person during Reiki share groups. I need to stress at this point that you can be awakened and attuned to Reiki after just one attunement. However, experience has shown me that students need time to digest progressively deeper attunements, as this allows gradual increases of energy and deeper levels of meditation. This period of attunement also enables a great amount of purification to take place and karma to be lifted.

Japanese Reiju Empowerments

Japanese *reiju* empowerments are the original Japanese form of attunements; Western attunements developed from *reiju* empowerments. The Japanese word *"reiju"* means "spiritual gift." *Reiju* empowerments are still being used today in Japan, although they vary according to the teacher. Whether the teacher uses a simple or complex method, the end result is that the student is opened and connected to Reiki for life.

I stopped using Western-style attunement after I received the knowledge and training of the *reiju* empowerments. I wanted to use methods that were closer to Mikao Usui's methods of teaching and to the Tendai Mikkyo Buddhist connections. The *reiju* empowerments were much more simple, more fluid, and easier to perform than the complicated Western attunement, so I could be much more relaxed in body and mind when giving the *reiju* empowerments. This created better empowerments for my students and for me. With the *reiju* empowerments, the Reiki teacher does not have to touch the student but places his or her hands in specific areas a couple of inches (five centimeters) away from the head, upper body, and hands. In a Western attunement, the teacher's hands touch the student.

During Western attunements, teachers use intention and the Reiki symbols, but during *reiju* empowerments, there are different options for awakening these qualities. A Reiki teacher may use the same empowerment over and over again during all the levels, using intention to define the level of empowerment. Another method is to chant one of the Reiki *kotodamas* during the process, in order to open the student to the quality of the *kotodama* mantra. In a *reiju* empowerment, the different energies aren't mixed; in contrast, in Western attunement, all Reiki energies may be used in one initiation. In Japan, Reiki students can receive a *reiju* empowerment as often as they wish, to help reinforce their connection and to help them along their spiritual path. Mikao Usui used to give *reiju* empowerments to his students simply by being in their presence, staring at them, and intending that they be awakened to Reiki. He did not have to touch them or undertake any rituals. In this way, Usui could open up many students to Reiki.

Distant Reiju Empowerment

If you live in a place or are in a situation where it is not easy, or even possible, for you to visit a Reiki teacher, there is another way of becoming initiated. You can be sent distant *reiju* empowerments to open your energy channels and connect you to Reiki.

This process is not a true substitute for learning Reiki from a Reiki teacher who is physically present, because he or she can't be there to support you and can't be responsible for any reaction that you may experience or for your actions during and after the empowerment. If you receive distant *reiju*, you must accept that you alone are responsible for the circumstances of your awakening; the teacher just sets up the method by which the Reiki will open you so that you can become a channel. It is your intention, your own open heart, and your desire to participate in the *reiju* that enable the connection to occur.

Anybody can receive a distant *reiju* empowerment both at the start of the process and at various times along the way. For example, I advise those of you who are already practicing Reiki to receive an empowerment daily or weekly to reinforce your connection to Reiki and help you on your spiritual path.

Receiving the Distant Reiju Empowerment

To receive the distant *reiju* empowerment, you should choose a time when you won't be interrupted and when you don't have anything pressing to do.

Instructions

1. Sit on a chair or on a cushion on the floor. If you are not able to leave your bed due to illness or disability, then receive the reiju empowerment from your bed.

2. Place your hands together into the prayer position at your heart. If this is not possible, then leave your hands on your lap or by your sides, palms facing up.

3. Ask for assistance from Reiki guides with this reiju empowerment.

4. Mentally intend that you receive the reiju empowerment. You may also say, "I am receiving the reiju empowerment from [teacher's name] now."

5. Let all thoughts come and go, and don't hang on to stray thoughts. Relax into the reiju empowerment and feel a gentle sensation fill you and wash over you.

6. When you wish to finish, think, "Reiju is ending now," and it will stop.

7. Place your hands palms down on your thighs or against your sides to maintain a connection and flow of the Reiki through your hands and channels.

8. Sit in silence for a moment and digest the Reiki.

9. Receive one reiju empowerment a day for four consecutive days. You may also receive the reiju empowerments over two days, one each morning and one each evening.

From this distant *reiju* connection, you will be connected to Reiki and you will be able to use it to heal yourself and your family and friends.

After Receiving All Four Distant Reiju Empowerments

After you have received the empowerments, it is advisable to give yourself Reiki for an hour a day for twenty-one days using the twelve basic hand positions. (I will show you these in chapter 5.) This allows you time to grow and to become accustomed to Reiki flowing through your channels and your body. The Reiki twenty-one-day cleanse will remove energy blockages in your channels that are causing you physical, mental, and emotional illness. It will make you a strong Reiki channel and a powerful soul. To perform the twenty-one-day Reiki cleanse, follow the instructions in chapter 6, "The Twenty-One-Day Cleanse."

Sensations and Experiences

Some students do not feel a great deal when receiving the *reiju* empowerment, while others encounter colors or light, internal heat, aches, and the surfacing of old pains and injuries of the body, mind, and heart. Common sensations are internal and external tingling, a dry throat, and feelings of peace.

Don't hold on to these sensations. Detach from them and watch them as though from a distance. Don't worry if you get cold or flu-like symptoms a day or so after the empowerment, because this is all quite normal, and it is evidence of the body responding to and adjusting to the energy that it is absorbing. The Reiki opens and unblocks energy channels in the body, and it so happens that cold and flu-like symptoms seem to be a natural reaction.

Grounding Yourself and Releasing Negativity

If you feel dizzy or nauseous after a *reiju* empowerment, focus your mind on the *hara* at your abdomen, just below the navel, and place both your palms on your abdomen. Breathe naturally while focusing on this area, and be aware of the abdomen gently moving in and out.

If you are still feeling a little ungrounded, move the point of focus to the center of the earth. Imagine a clear white light coming from heaven, entering your body through the crown of your head and washing through you, so that it washes a cloud of darkness or murky water through you, and out through your feet and into the earth. Maintain your awareness in the earth until you feel comfortable.

This grounding method may also be used if you feel you are receiving negativity from another person after giving a treatment.

It can also be useful if you are on the receiving end of other people's careless thoughts. If you want to release heavy negative energies from yourself, do so when the phase of the moon is new or full, as these are "power times" that make it easy for you to receive large quantities of spiritual energy and also to rid yourself of negativity. You can also ground yourself by eating some food, going for a walk, or getting some fresh air.

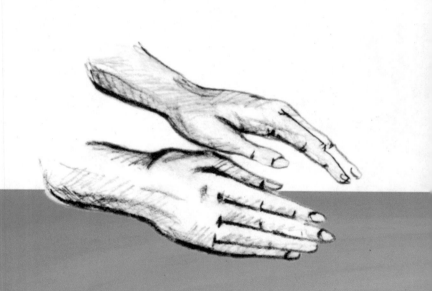

The Twelve Basic Hand Positions for Self-Healing

5

There are twelve basic hand positions for treating the mind, body, and emotions; students are taught these positions at the first level of Reiki. It is said that Usui taught only five positions, which were focused around the head, and that he used intuition to treat the rest of the body. A student of Usui's, Dr. Chujiro Hayashi, built upon the original system and created the system of twelve hand positions. Hayashi researched and created structured hand positions that focused on specific energy points around the body. This method of treatment was more holistic, affecting not only the body, but also the mind and emotions, even when they weren't the focus of the treatment.

Hawayo Takata introduced the twelve basic Reiki hand positions to the West. These positions can be used to treat stress, back pain, headache, arthritis, skin problems such as eczema, insomnia, irritable bowel syndrome, inflammation and swelling, depression, mental and emotional imbalance, fears, and many other maladies. With prolonged treatment, a sense of inner strength and peace grows in the affected person. In turn, this enables the body, emotions, and mind to rejuvenate and to develop a sense of space and calm. If you give yourself regular Reiki treatments, a feeling of peace will grow within you. This should help you to view circumstances more positively and with love and detachment.

You will use these twelve hand positions in the twenty-one-day cleanse, described in the next chapter. Remember the twelve basic healing positions by breaking them down into three parts.

Part 1: Four head positions
Part 2: Four front positions
Part 3: Four back positions

The Four Head Positions

Position 1: Eyes and Cheeks

Place your cupped hands over your eyes, cheeks, and forehead, and hold this position for five minutes. This will treat the associated areas of eyes, nose, cheeks, brain, the upper energy center, and the energy points around the same areas. It may relieve sinus problems, congestion from colds, eye infections, and headaches. It will help to make your mind clearer so that you can focus and concentrate.

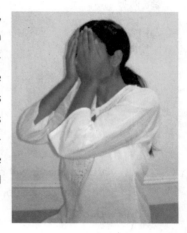

Position 2: Temples and Spiritual Eye

Place your hands over your temples and hold them there for five minutes. This will treat the associated areas of the temples, eyes, ears, brain, and glands within those areas. It may relieve an overactive mind, tension, depression, insomnia, headaches, and eye and ear problems. Both hemispheres of the brain are energetically balanced. This position will calm the mind. Over the next few days, you may notice your dreams more, and this may bother you

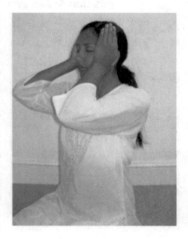

for a while, but this effect will soon fade away and your dreams will return to their normal pattern.

Position 3: Base of the Skull

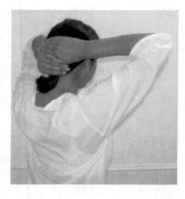

Place your hands at the base of your skull where your neck and skull meet, and hold this position for five minutes. The entire nervous system is connected via the head and neck through the spine.

This position calms and rejuvenates the nervous system, so this is a very relaxing position. It treats the skull, neck, eyes, nose, mouth, and both hemispheres of the brain. It also treats many parts of the body via the spine. It will relieve stress, nervousness, tension, headaches, and congestion, and it enriches the energy center at the back of the head.

Position 4: Jaw and Throat

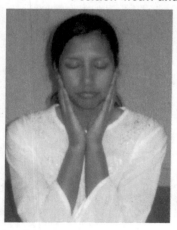

Gently rest your hands along your jawline, with the bases of your palms touching each other and resting over your throat. This position treats your jaw, mouth, teeth and gums, neck, larynx, and throat. It may relieve a sore throat, toothache, and jaw ache. It may release emotions and allow you to get things that have been suppressed off your chest, and it enriches the energy center at the throat.

The Four Front Positions

Position 5: Heart and Chest

Place your hands over your heart at the center of your chest or breastbone. This position treats the heart, chest, breast, rib cage, lungs, shoulders, hands, and arms. It also treats the spiritual energy center of the heart. (You may know this area as the heart chakra.) This center connects you to your true self, moving you away from your ego and allowing you to experience the lightness and true love of the soul. You can move your hands around the whole of the chest and breast area using this position.

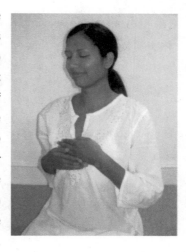

It can relieve breathing problems and treat stress, insomnia, and depression. It can induce relaxation, calm, and peace. Suppressed emotions associated with self-dislike and hatred of others can be awakened, released, and accepted, creating a feeling of spaciousness and peace. This will bring you into a state of balance and harmony. It has been reported that many people fall asleep at this point!

Position 6: Stomach and Solar Plexus

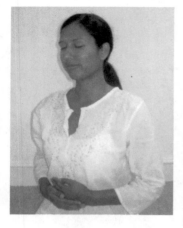

Place your hands on your stomach and solar plexus. This position treats the stomach, liver, spleen, diaphragm, intestines, and bowels. It can relieve digestive illness, ulcers, stomachache, and nervous conditions. The solar plexus is a creative-feeling energy center, in which you experience stress, fear, and tension, so healing this position brings relief to emotional stress and anger. Treating this area can release and relieve many emotions that may be causing the associated organs to suffer. With prolonged treatment of this area, the emotions become balanced, so you will feel more confident and more aligned with your heart's desires.

Position 7: Navel and Upper Abdomen

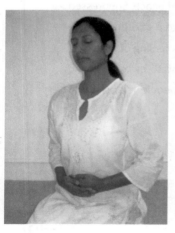

Place your hands over and just below your navel on your upper abdomen. This position treats the kidneys, gall bladder, appendix, pelvis, ovaries, and gonads. It may relieve kidney and bladder infections, abdominal cramps, bloating, menstrual pains, and constipation. The lower energy center, known as the *hara*, is seated at this position; great quantities of energy can be stored here, and many energetic channels meet and cross here as well. There are methods within Reiki that focus solely on this area to bring health and spirituality.

Position 8: Lower Abdomen and Pelvis

Place your hands over your lower abdomen, below where they

were in position 7. In this position also, there is space to move your hands around your abdomen and at the sides of your pelvis. This position treats the bladder, genitals, colon, anus, prostate gland, ovaries, pelvis, and hips. It may relieve hip pains and stiffness, bladder infections, hemorrhoid pain, bloating, menstrual pains, and abdominal cramps. When this area is being treated, childhood memories and suppressed emotions related to family and 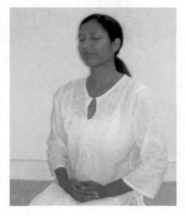 friends may surface. The base energy center at the perineum and the second energy center at the base of the spine are treated and enriched with Reiki.

The Four Back Positions

Position 9: Upper Back and Shoulders

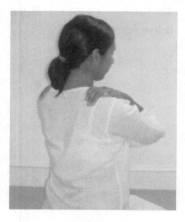

Place your hands on your shoulders and your upper back. This position treats the neck, shoulders, spine, upper back, heart, and lungs. It may relieve shoulder, neck, and upper back pain, knots, tension, and stress. Its effects are similar to those of position 5, heart and chest (one of the four front positions). However, while you work on this position, Reiki also enriches and treats smaller energy channels and points that exist in the shoulders and upper back.

Position 10: Shoulders and Shoulder Blades

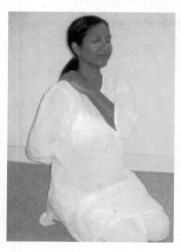

Position 10 is the trickiest of the twelve, as it involves some flexibility. It is best to be as relaxed as possible when holding this position and to go only as far as your body allows you to without discomfort. Position 10 is also split into two parts, so that both shoulder blades are treated. This means holding the position for two and a half minutes on each shoulder blade, for a total of five minutes.

If you find this position difficult, you may turn over the hand that is around your

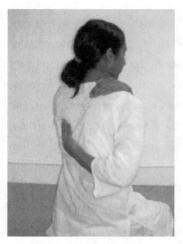

back so that your palm is facing away from your shoulder blade until you are used to holding your arm and hand in this position. This will relieve some of the pressure in the shoulder, elbow, and wrist.

Position 11: Lower Back

Place your hands over your lower back. This position treats the lower back, kidneys, bladder, lower spine, intestines, bowels, spleen, liver, and ovaries. It can relieve menstrual pains, cramps, sciatica, stress, and tension in the back, lower spine, and discs. In fact, it can relieve all kinds of back pain. A very important, circular energy channel runs around the waist, connecting at this point with many other energy channels. A center point for this channel is at the middle of the spine at the lower back between the kidneys.

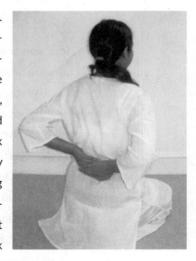

Position 12: Base of the Spine

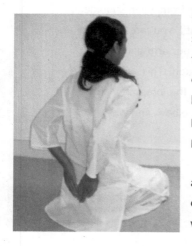

Place your hands over the base of your spine at your buttocks. This position treats the coccyx, buttocks, genitals, kidneys, colon, rectum, bladder, prostate, pelvis, and legs. It may relieve sciatica, hemorrhoid pain, bladder infections, colon and rectum pain, and lower back and spinal pain.

Past childhood memories and emotions associated with families, friends, and associates may be released, relieved, and let go while the base energy center is treated.

• • •

You may treat your arms, hands, legs, and feet if you wish, though this will take you beyond the twelve basic positions and will add to the hour that you are already spending on your self-healing. The twelve positions are a guideline and the foundation for treating yourself and others. As you progress, you will let go of the mental, emotional, and intellectual constraints that are making you sick. Eventually, you will move beyond the twelve positions, letting Reiki guide you with intuition, love, and an open heart.

What does it mean to allow Reiki to guide you? Simply this: at some time in the future, you will no longer stick rigidly to every one of the recommended hand positions. You will certainly do most, if not all, of them, but then you will move on to the bodily areas that most need your attention. You won't need to ask your client about this, because the Reiki itself will make you so in tune with the needs of your client that it will take your hands to the place where the healing is most needed. Oddly enough, you may not be drawn to the exact point where the person is hurting but to a place where the healing can do the most good.

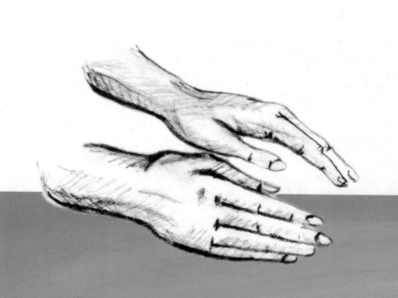

The
Twenty-One-Day
Cleanse

6

During the twenty-one-day cleanse, you spend one hour a day treating yourself. Over the course of this hour, you use each of the twelve self-treatment hand positions, holding each position for five minutes. You can break this daily treatment up into two half-hour sessions, one in the morning and the one in the evening, doing the first six hand positions in the morning and the rest later in the day.

The twenty-one-day cleanse may bring on cold or flu-like symptoms, or you may feel emotionally or mentally off balance, up and down, with moments of happiness and sadness, peace, bliss, laughing, and crying. You may feel sensations of heat and cold, a dry mouth, heaviness, dense sensations in the head, tingling, or aches and pains. Old memories, habits, and behavior patterns that you have suppressed may reemerge.

It's important to take a detached view of the symptoms and continue with the cleanse, even if it is mentally or physically uncomfortable, because this shows that you are accumulating the spiritual energy that will give you the strength to deal with your symptoms. If you stop the practice because you believe that Reiki is making you feel ill or unhappy, you will become stuck in the old pattern of emotion, pain, depression, or whatever else was making you ill. Reiki is the catalyst that will lead you to integration and freedom, and to love and peace. When you make the choice to tread the spiritual path, you must keep your motivation going, and you must work hard at it. Be kind to yourself and to others, and listen to your heart, while tuning out your mind and the reaction of your emotions. The heart is the gateway to your soul.

Drink a few glasses of water a day during this process, as this will help to rid the body of dead cells and toxins. Be aware that this practice tends to increase bowel movements and the passing of urine as well.

Treating Yourself Using the Twelve Basic Hand Positions

You can practice the twelve basic hand positions while sitting on a chair or lying down, as long as you are flexible enough to do the back positions.

It is best to practice in peace and quiet or with some relaxing music in the background. Technically, you could do these positions while watching television, but I don't recommend it, as it is better to be relaxed and to concentrate on the treatment.

- To begin, mentally affirm, "Reiki is starting now."

- You may mentally invoke help from Reiki guides, spiritual guides, angels, gods, goddesses, and other deities, or you can ask the guidance of Reiki itself.

- Have a glass of water available and keep a clock handy so that you can keep track of the time.

- Place the fingers and thumbs together on each hand; then gently cup the hands slightly. This will help to focus the energy into the palms rather than spreading the energy outward. Hold each hand position for five minutes.

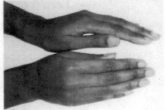

Each hand position treats the area where the hands are placed, including the organs below the surface of the skin. Reiki also travels to areas that require healing, which may be an area that is affecting you mentally or emotionally, or something physical that you are unaware of. When an area of energy becomes unblocked, there may be a brief release in the form of pain, a popping and bubbling sensation followed by laughing or crying, and finally a feeling of calm.

Not everybody encounters these symptoms, and those who do encounter them usually find them to be mild. Symptoms are part of the creative force of Reiki healing.

Handy Tips

- It's best to practice in peace.

- Have a clock and a glass of water available.

- Listen to Reiki music or other relaxing music. Do all twelve positions sitting or lying down. Hold each position for five minutes.

- Mentally ask for help for your treatment from Reiki, Usui, and your Reiki guides.

- Keep your fingers together and your hands slightly cupped during the treatment.

- Finish by saying, "Reiki is ending now."

- Give thanks to your Reiki guides, Reiki, and Usui.

- Keep a journal of your feelings and experiences, as this can be useful for future reference.

Reasons for Doing the Cleanse

Why is it so important to do the twenty-one-day cleanse? The effort involved is a bit like that involved in visiting a wonderful holiday resort in a mountainous area a long way from where you live. You must pack everything up, put all the luggage and things you will need in the car, and get the kids ready and into the car. Then you drive for hours, keeping the children amused the best you can. The last part of the journey takes you higher and higher through increasingly beautiful countryside, until you reach your wonderful destination. Needless to say, it's worth it when you get there. Likewise, the preparation and onset of the Reiki journey will involve some work on your part, but when you reach your "destination" of achieving the twenty-one-day cleanse, the effort expended will definitely seem worthwhile.

While a book like this can explain the art of Reiki, in the end becoming proficient at Reiki is like learning to drive or use a computer. A book will help you learn to do all of these things, but it can't actually do the job for you. You can't expect to treat and heal others until you have "cleansed" yourself, and you can't expect to prepare yourself for Reiki without giving up a little of your spare time. When you consider how long it takes to train for many other things in life, expending a little time each day for three weeks is not a big deal. Always keep in mind: your awareness and understanding of Reiki will increase as each day goes by.

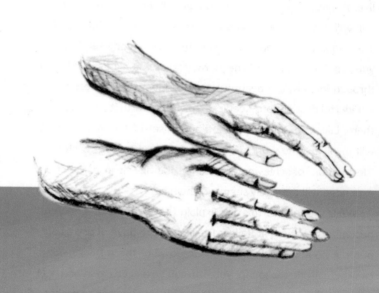

Giving
Reiki
Treatments
to Others

7

Once you have completed the twenty-one-day cleanse, you will be ready to try out your healing ability on others. Treating your family, friends, and loved ones is a good way to gain experience, get feedback, and get an honest opinion. This will make you more confident, and it will make your Reiki stronger as well.

Not only does Reiki address the ailment of the person being treated; it also treats the healer at the same time. A healer benefits from divine healing and comfort regardless of how accomplished he or she might be. Healers tend to be people who have suffered a lot in their own lives, and while this is what makes them great healers, it also makes them need divine help and healing. This makes Reiki a win-win situation, because it aids both the recipient of the healing and the healer at the same time.

Giving a Reiki treatment to others using the twelve basic hand positions is similar to giving yourself a one-hour treatment. If you have done the twenty-one-day Reiki cleanse on yourself, then you should find giving a treatment to somebody else relatively simple.

Most people understand a little about Reiki and other forms of mind, body, and spirit healing, and they know that Reiki's methods are quiet, respectful, subdued, and genteel. If you have relatives or friends who you think could benefit from Reiki, tell them about it, but don't force the issue. If they decide that they would like your help, they will ask for it.

Once you have a willing subject to practice on, give your friend a full-body treatment using the twelve hand positions. If it isn't possible to have your subject lie down, give the treatment while he or she is sitting in a chair. You may use the twelve hand positions, but you may have to adapt them to reach the required areas of the body while your subject is sitting. Giving a treatment to a seated person allows you to treat the front and back areas more quickly, speeding up the treatment. The sitting version of treatment can be done anywhere, but using a bed or treatment table allows your patient to get maximum relaxation, which definitely benefits your patient.

Never pressure people into having a treatment. Their minds will block it out and they won't get any benefit from it. Giving and receiving Reiki require an open heart and an open mind, so leave those who are closed off or self-protective to their own devices.

Should You Treat Strangers?

If you intend to treat strangers, with or without payment, you must consider your position. There are many independent Reiki healers who have no special qualifications or affiliations to any organization, and they are probably very good at what they do, but in Europe, they are in breach of European Union regulations, and elsewhere, similar problems may arise. You must carry public liability and other insurance. In the United States, it is essential that you be insured. There are insurers who will cover complementary therapists and Reiki healers, and a search through the Internet will locate them. It is your responsibility to be aware of the legal requirements in your country.

It is equally important that you join a professional body of Reiki teachers and students and become certified and qualified.

This way, you will gain the supervised experience necessary to be able to handle all the possible problems that can arise from time to time—remember, you are dealing with people, not toys. If you don't know where to find these organizations, try searching the Internet. Simply reading this book will not qualify you as a Reiki practitioner; this book is meant to introduce you to the physical and spiritual benefits of treating yourself.

The Treatment Room

Your treatment room should be free of clutter. It should be quiet, light, and warm, and it should have fresh air and good air circulation, if possible. This will enable a free flow of energy around the room and will make the environment much more conducive to healing. Spaces for rent in clinics or therapy centers are usually suitable. It may be helpful to play some relaxing music, but it isn't a good idea to light incense. Incense can have a very powerful effect on the senses; it can make some people cough; and not everybody likes the smell. If you choose to use incense, light it a few hours before starting to work, as it will purify the energy and air in the room but the smell will have a chance to disperse before the treatment begins.

Treatment Preparations

If you are going to do more than the occasional treatment for friends, you will need to buy a treatment table or you will need to rent space in a center where a table is available. As mentioned earlier, you can give a Reiki treatment to a seated person when necessary. I have used this method of treatment with great success at healing exhibitions and for family and friends. However, when you give a one-hour treatment, I recommend that you use a treatment table with the patient lying down, so that he or she benefits from maximum relaxation, as this will help the treatment. Trying to heal someone who is lying on the floor is uncomfortable for both Reiki practitioner and subject.

You need to be able to sit and talk with your patients before you start treatment. You may want to know what is wrong with them and what has prompted them to seek treatment. You will certainly want to take notes and to keep a record of their details. You will need an appointment book or a date book for making and recording appointments.

Keep a bottle of water and some paper cups handy, because the treatment will make both you and your patients thirsty. Water will help the process of the healing. After a Reiki treatment, the energy purifies the body by increasing the removal of bodily waste through urination and bowel movements. This is why it is

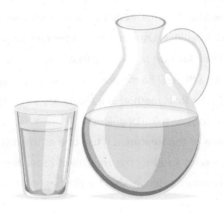

advisable to recommend to the person receiving the treatment to avoid alcohol and heavy meals the night before and on the day of the treatment.

Have tissues available, because a Reiki treatment helps blocked emotions, pain, and memories to gradually be released and accepted. Your client may react to the treatment with tears, physical pain, or happiness. If emotions surface during the treatment, ask your patient if he or she wishes to stop briefly, and offer tissues and a drink of water. Above all, let your patient know that this is a normal and temporary response to Reiki healing.

You need a clock where you can see it easily, so that you can keep to your schedule.

You may want to have a pillow and a blanket available for your patients, as lying still for an hour during the treatment may make them feel cold. It is often more comfortable for them to have their heads on a pillow.

Starting a Treatment

Before I give a treatment, I mentally ask for assistance and protection from Reiki guides, Usui, and the divine energy of Reiki itself. I ask that I not take on any karma from the people I am giving healing to. Use the *reiji hô* method by mentally asking those who worked with the Reiki method in its early days, including Usui, to connect you to your spiritual guides.

In advance of the treatment, I use one of the distant-healing methods to send Reiki to the treatment room for me and for the person being treated, asking for the best outcome from the session. The best outcome of a healing session isn't necessarily what you or the recipient would want for the healing, but is sometimes what is needed for the recipient's (and your) learning and spiritual path.

Byosen: Scanning the Body for Illness

Again, use the *reiji hô* by mentally asking the originators of the Reiki method, including Usui, to connect you to your spiritual guides. Ask Reiki to guide your hands to areas that need healing. In this way, your hands become like magnets, and they are drawn to specific vibrations and sensations on the body of the patient. This scanning method is called *"byosen."* It will help you to identify areas in the patient's body and energy field that may be unbalanced or have an energetic block in the energy channel that is causing some dysfunction.

Starting above the crown of your client's head, very slowly and gently sweep your hands down through his or her energy field, with your hands about four or five inches (ten centimeters) away from the person's body. Keep your fingers and thumbs together during this process, and move very slowly from head to toe once or twice, if you have the time. When you return to the person's head, keep an energetic connection by leaving your hand in the person's energy field. You are trying to become aware of any area and sensation that your hands are being drawn to. These sensations will help you access the areas that require healing.

Cold

A very cold sensation being projected from an area in the body or energy field into your palms is an indication of an energy blockage. The cold area usually indicates a deep-rooted emotional or spiritual problem, which may be causing a physical reaction. This will need a lot of healing, which will take time, because the root of the blockage may not be obvious. You may need to mentally ask your guides to send healing energy to the client in order to relieve the pain that is lingering within the client as a result of past hurts.

Giving a treatment using all the twelve hand positions is a good way of treating deep-rooted problems, because the mind and emotions are helped during this kind of treatment. It is an effective and gentle way of healing the whole person.

Heat

A great deal of heat coming from some part of your patient suggests one of two things. It can indicate an excess of energy in this area, and you can ease this by placing your hands on and around the hot area. It can also mean that great amounts of Reiki are being poured into the area and starting the healing process on a badly damaged body part or energy field. Heat usually indicates a physical problem rather than an emotional problem.

Tingling

If you feel tingling and slight pain in your hands when you hold them over a particular part of your patient, this may indicate deep skin and cell damage caused by scarring or spinal injections, such as epidurals or other local anesthetic treatments that have been put into the spinal shaft. It can also denote some form of anger that is affecting a body part.

Denseness

Your hands may feel heavy and slow as they travel through an area, as though they are moving through molasses. The dense area is where the energy has become sluggish; this sluggishness can be due to depression or mental or emotional illness. Giving a whole-body treatment can bring this energy to the surface, where you can sweep it out from the energy field, leaving the patient with a feeling of lightness. You do this by placing a bowl of salt at the foot of the treatment couch. Then you sweep your hands over the client's body from head to toe, without actually touching him or her. The negative energies that you have brought up into the client's aura can now be swept away from the client and down into the bowl of salt. Remove the salt bowl, and then later you wash the salt away down the drain.

Vibration

If your hands vibrate or if the patient feels as though he or she is vibrating during or after the treatment, this signifies the removal of energy blockages or a purifying of the energy channels and centers. Powerful energy may be working through the patient's system to balance and rejuvenate their energy channels. Another feature of this symptom is that the patient (and sometimes also the healer) will receive even more healing later when asleep.

Magnetic Pull

If your hands are drawn to an area as if a magnet is pulling them there, leave them in the area until the sensation subsides. This signifies an area that needs healing.

Pain

Sometimes you may feel the pain of the person you are treating. This happens when a highly positively charged vibration comes into contact with a highly negatively charged vibration. You become a little like a syringe sucking out the poison. If the pain bothers you, break contact for a moment. If you maintain your position, staying with the pain, it will soon subside. If it continues, call upon your Reiki guides and Usui, asking them to take this karma and illness from you. You are doing your job, and they must do theirs when called upon. Remember to also ask for this negative energy to be removed from you after you have finished your healing session.

Visual Impressions

Your intuition and spiritual eye can become much stronger when practicing Reiki, and you may notice this increased strength during treatments. A person may simply stand before you, and you may pick up an impression from his or her energy field. This impression can be symbolic or literal, and it will be different for each person. On one occasion, I saw darkness in the lungs of a person, and at first I was uncertain why. The mind has a tendency to jump to conclusions when this happens, so it is not always best to share the information with the person you are healing, as it may scare them. On this occasion, the blackness of the lungs was showing me that this person was suffering because of smoking. The impressions you get, even those that appear to be negative, do not always mean that the person is ill, but in this example, the person was trying to give up smoking, which was one of the reasons the person had come for a treatment.

Not every Reiki healer feels things in the same way, so the feelings that I have described are only a guide to what might happen. In time, you'll discover your own triggers and indicators. Experience is a great teacher.

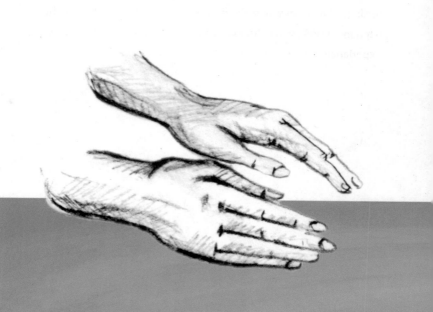

The Twelve Basic Hand Positions for Healing Others

8

H ere are some useful tips to bear in mind before you start to use the twelve basic hand positions for healing:

- Hold your hands in each position for five minutes.

- Staying still for five minutes is quite difficult, so make sure you are comfortable. This is why sitting on a chair can be helpful while you are doing the head positions.

- Refer to the chapter on treating yourself (chapter 6) to discover what each hand position treats.

- To intensify the Reiki in certain areas on the body when you are giving a treatment, simply place one hand on top of the other.

- If your client has a sensitive area on his or her body, or if he or she has an open wound such as an ulcer, then hold your hand above the area and focus Reiki energy on the wound, rather than touching it.

The Four Head Positions

Position 1: Eyes and Cheeks

With your client either sitting or standing, gently place your hands over your client's eyes and cheeks. Do not cover your client's nose as you may impede his or her breathing. Remember not to put too much pressure on your client's face,

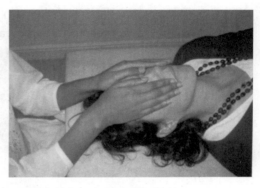

especially if you are standing, as you may find yourself leaning without realizing it.

Position 2: Temples and Spiritual Eye

Place your hands on both temples with your thumbs touching the patient's spiritual eye.

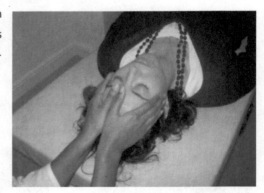

Position 3: Back of the Head

This position can be quite tricky, so it is advisable to show your client what you are going to do before you start your treatment. This way, your client may help you by lifting his or her head slightly so you may get your hands underneath.

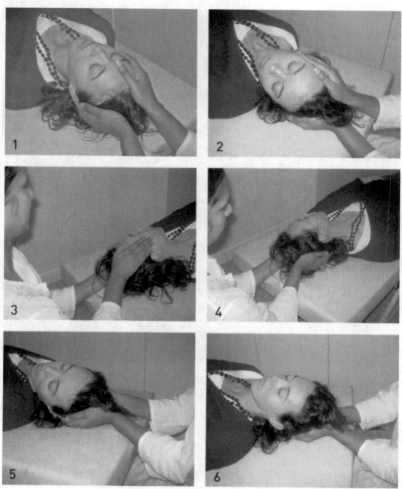

Start this position where the last position ends.

1. Keep your right hand on the patient's right temple and gently slide your left hand down as far as possible under the back of the client's head.

2. With your right hand on the right temple, gently turn and move the client's head to the left, sliding the head onto your left hand.

3. With the head turned to the left, slide your right hand down under the back of the head.

4. Both hands should now be side by side under the back of your client's head.

5. With both of your hands gently cupping the back of the head, move the head back to the center.

6. You are now in the third hand-healing position.

7. To remove your hands from this position, follow the same procedure, starting from the back of the head and following the instructions in reverse order.

Position 4: Jaw and Throat

Before you start your treatment with position 4 (see page 76), tell your client you are going place your hands close to his or her neck, because this is a vulnerable area that may invoke insecurities.

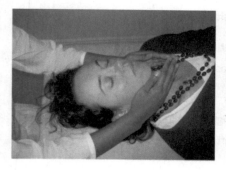

Gently place your hands on both sides of your client's jawline so your hands also cover the throat. Your fingers on both hands should meet over your client's throat, creating a V shape.

The Four Front Positions

Position 5: Heart and Chest

If you are seated, you can reach over gently from the last position and lay your hands on the center of the patient's chest. This central point is where the heart energy center is located. If you are standing, you should place your hands side by side, but you can also move your hands to any area of the chest if you have enough time.

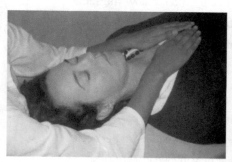

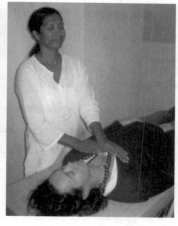

Position 6: Stomach and Solar Plexus

Gently place your hands on the solar plexus and stomach area. This area is located between the chest and the navel. Treat the central point, then move your hands around the area. You may put your hands side by side or one in front of the other when treating this area.

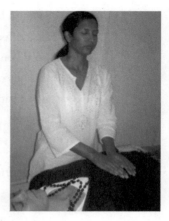

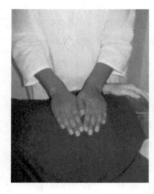

Position 7: Navel and Upper Abdomen

Place your hands onto your client's upper abdomen with your hands one in front of the other.

Position 8: Lower Abdomen and Pelvis

Place your hands on the lower abdomen, just below the last position.

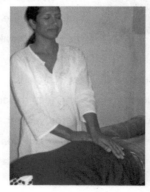

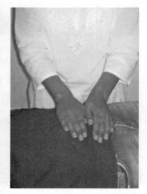

You can finish by sending Reiki to either the front or the back of the legs and feet. Working down the legs, knees, and feet is optional, so if you are short of time, it is a good idea to simply place your hands on both sides of the legs and work down them, holding each position for a few seconds until you reach the feet. Hold your hands above the client's feet if you do not wish to touch them, and send Reiki onto them from that position.

Sweeping the Energy Field

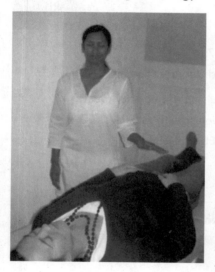

Now you must use your hands to sweep the energy field, while also using your mind to visualize all dark energies leaving your client's energy field. The dark energy is said to come to the surface of the energy field during a treatment. A good way to visualize this is to imagine looking into some clear water and then gently swirling your hand around in the pool. The swirling motion brings all the sediment at the bottom of the pool to the surface, making the water appear murky. Sweeping the energy field removes the sediment that comes to the surface during a treatment.

The movements you use to sweep the energy field look a little like those used in tai chi. The movement of your hands is soft, fluid, and relaxed, with gentle force that comes as much from your mind as anything. Your body, legs, arms, hands, and mind all have to work in unity.

Move your hands from the last treatment position at your client's feet to above the crown of his or her head while still keeping your hands in your client's energy field.

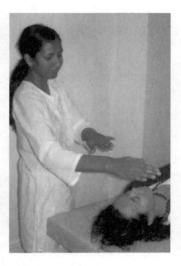

Stand to the side of your client and place your hands one in front of the other about eight inches (twenty centimeters) above your client, in his or her energy field.

Imagine that both your hands are gently locked together in this position, so that when one hand moves, the other moves in harmony with it. If you don't do this, you may be uncomfortable while performing this action.

Slightly tilt your hands at a forty-degree angle, using just your wrists. This way, you will catch and push the dark cloud of energy out of your client's energy field using your palms and fingers.

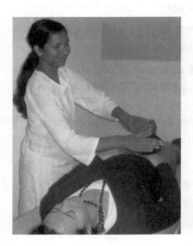

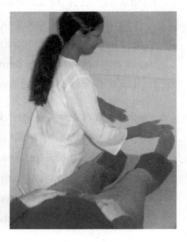

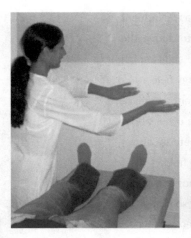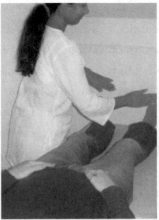

Gently move your hands forward in a circular motion through your client's energy field while visualizing a buildup of black cloud being gathered in front of your hands, leaving behind it a light, vibrant energy field. Move your hands in a small circular motion to enable you to cover a larger area in the energy field. Your second hand will go over the same area again, to ensure that it is clear.

Sweep the black cloud down to the client's feet, and then make a large sweeping motion with your hands. Feel and visualize the black cloud of energy being swept out of your client's energy field, and in your mind see it dissolving into a brilliant light.

Note: Spiritual healers don't like throwing detritus of this kind around a room, so they put a bowl with a little salt in it on the floor, and they throw the dark energy into it. (Salt draws out bad vibes and energies and destroys them.) After treating a few clients, and as soon as it is convenient, they wash the salt down the drain and then replenish the bowl with fresh salt.

The Four Back Positions

Gently support your client with one hand and ask him or her to turn over.

Scanning the Body

Before treating the back and legs, you may want to quickly scan the client's body again if you have the time. This will give you an idea of areas that may require more or less intensive treatment.

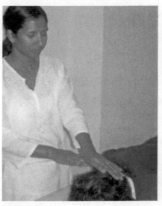
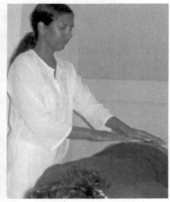

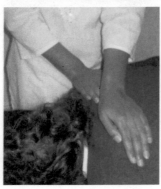

Position 9: Upper Back and Shoulders

You may sit or stand while doing treatment with this position. Lay your hands on the client's shoulders and around his or her upper back.

Position 10: Shoulders and Shoulder Blades

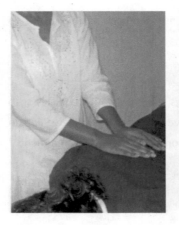 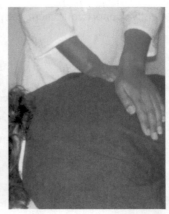

Lay your hands on the area of the shoulder blades. You can also treat the upper area of the back with this position.

Position 11: Lower Back

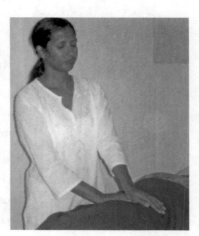

Lay your hands either side by side or one in front of the other on the lower back. Many people suffer from lower back pain, so this can be quite a comforting area to treat.

Position 12: Base of Spine

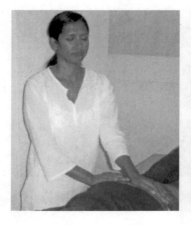 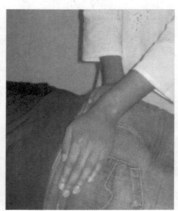

Lay your hands on the base of the spine. You may treat around the buttock area and hips with this position.

Bringing Energy up the Spine

From the last position, place one hand in front of the other, starting at the base of the spine. Hold each position for about five seconds, gently moving both hands up the spine as if they were stuck together.

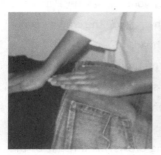 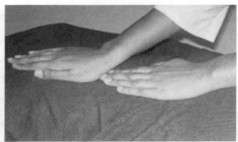

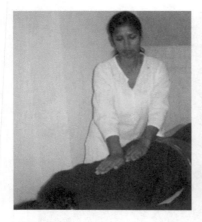
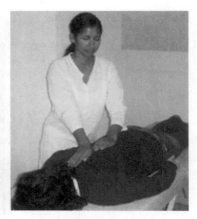

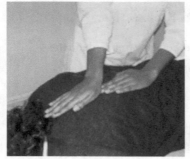
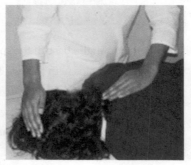

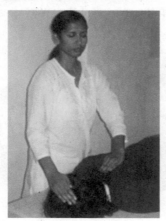

This action should finish with one hand on your client's neck and the other on or above the crown of your client's head.

This method gently brings energy up the spine to the head. This will help refresh and awaken a client who has fallen asleep, or one who is feeling drowsy as a result of the Reiki treatment.

Sweeping the Back Energy Field

Finish the Reiki treatment by sweeping the energy field on the back of the body, exactly as you did for the front of the body.

After Giving a Treatment

Keep one hand on your client to make sure he or she doesn't fall off the table, and gently let your client know that the treatment is finished. Offer your client a glass of water, as the treatment usually makes the throat and mouth dry. Inform your client that the energy will be working through him or her for the next few days and that he or she should drink water to aid purification.

Inform your client that if he or she feels a little low or out of balance during the next few days, this is a normal response to the treatment because dissipating blocked energy can lead to emotional or physical reactions. This is all part of the healing process.

Ask your client how he or she felt during the treatment, and if he or she is feeling better or worse in areas that may have been addressed during the treatment. Take notes about how your client is feeling, and also note down what you did for your client during the treatment. I was taught that it takes three consecutive treatments to benefit from receiving Reiki because it is cumulative and needs to build up over the course of time to be really effective.

Most important, spend a minute or so by yourself after the treatment using the *reiji hô* method to connect to Reiki, Reiki guides, and Usui. Ask them to remove and wash away any negativity or strange energies that you may have taken on from your client during the treatment.

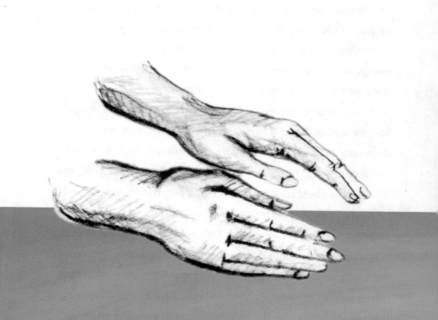

Mikao Usui's Reiki Treatments

9

We know that Usui's methods for giving treatments were more open, fluid, and intuitively guided than the somewhat formal methods that Western Reiki masters teach. Like many other kinds of spiritual healers, Usui relied on the universe for help and guidance. His teaching method reflected this openness, so he gave different suggestions regarding methods to different students, depending on their intuition, openness to guidance, and awareness of spiritual energy.

Usui used five head positions rather than full-body positions; you might want to try these as an experiment. Use these positions as a starting point, and then allow spiritual guidance to move your hands into areas on your own body that Reiki wants to heal. You can even sit perfectly still and use nothing other than meditation to visualize your hands treating any area of your body. See if you

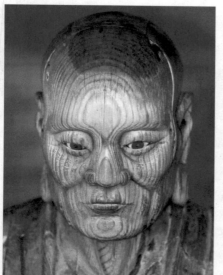

can feel the flow of Reiki from your subtle plane to your physical body.

Usui's five special hand positions are related to the Bodhisattva Binzuru, who was a senior disciple to Buddha and who was well known for his healing abilities. Each one of these hand positions is a mudra (seal of energy) of Binzuru. It is said that placing our hands in these mudras invokes the healing powers of Binzuru on an unconscious level.

Usui's Five Original Hand Positions

1. Kneel down in the *seiza* position (leaving about two hands' width between your knees). Your weight should be evenly distributed on your buttocks, and not too far back or forward on your legs; alternatively, you can sit on a chair.

2. Start at the head, using the following five hand positions and holding each one for at least five minutes.

3. All energy channels converge from your head through your body, so by treating your head, you can receive a full body healing.

4. When you have completed the head treatment, use your intuition to treat other parts of your body. Use the *reiji hô* method to increase your intuitive guidance.

Five Healing Positions

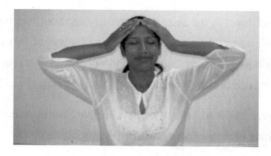

Zentô bu: The top of your forehead at the start of your hairline

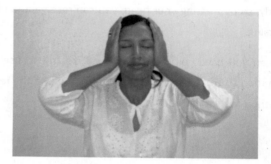

Sokutô bu: Both sides of your head at your temples

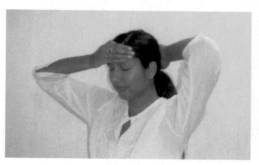

Kôtô bu: Your forehead and the upper back of your skull;
treat both areas at the same time

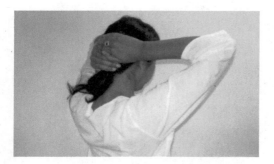

Enzui bu: The back of your head where your spine and skull meet

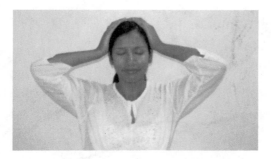

Tôchô bu: The top of your head at the crown

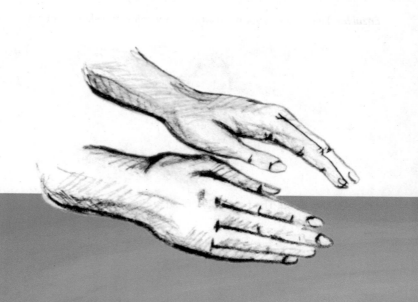

The First Degree of Reiki: Shoden

10

There are three levels of Reiki, which we in the West call degrees. In addition, there is a fourth degree for potential teachers. Each degree allows you to receive deeper knowledge and methods for healing and spiritual awareness, giving you a foundation to work with as the style of Reiki unfolds. It also allows you time to appreciate what you have learned in each degree segment, and each degree gives you a taste for the other levels as you progress.

In Japan, first-degree Reiki was referred to as *shoden*, which means "beginning level." This is the introduction and awakening of Reiki channels for the student. Usui's methods focused on the students being awakened to Reiki through many *reiju* empowerments. It is the empowerment that opens and creates a channel that connects you to Reiki. Once you have received the empowerments, you will be given specific methods that reinforce your connection and allow you to cultivate the Reiki. This level is about purification, self-healing, and instruction in the basics of healing.

In the West, this first Reiki level is generally taught over two days with around ten to twelve hours' training. When I teach, I use practices that are taken directly from the Japanese origins and that tap into the mystic traditions of Japan, but I also use a Western approach to make it more accessible to my students.

Opening Your Heart

It is important to open your heart and soul to Usui, Reiki, and the source of Reiki.

The lineage of Reiki refers to those who first discovered and developed the system. By mentally linking with them, you start to build a relationship that melts blocks in your heart and allows the energy, healing, and intuitive guidance to flow through you powerfully and clearly. It is important to build a relationship with Reiki, Usui, and the source of Reiki, as this will open you up to higher energies, and to peace, bliss, and the spiritually intuitive guidance that will take you beyond the confines of the mind. Before a meditation or before giving a Reiki treatment, ask for assistance from the Reiki lineage to help bring the highest energies through you to allow you to heal the person who has asked for your help. You will come to understand that *you* are not doing the healing; instead, the lineage and source work through you once you surrender to their love, light, and grace.

I was taught that Reiki protects healers while they are giving treatments; in this way, they don't take on the karmas of their patients during or after the treatment. Some of my students and I are sensitive to the energies of some of our patients, so we feel and experience their physical and emotional pain during and for some time after a treatment. This does eventually pass, but I recommend that you remove it right away. Connect to the lineage, Usui, Buddha, and Reiki because this connection dilutes and diffuses the karmas that we are in touch with during and after treatments. I suggest that you make this connection at the end of every treatment. For a few minutes, mentally ask and pray for Reiki to remove any of your patient's energies from you. If a few minutes are not enough, continue to connect until you feel better.

Protecting Yourself

You should try to practice this meditation every day. When you have finished meditating, mentally request that your own problems and stresses be relieved. If you have questions or problems of your own, ask for answers to be sent to you.

Although this may seem as though you are just saying a few simple words, in fact you are pointing the direction of your soul and heart toward the Reiki lineage and invoking the help and guidance that you need. If you build a relationship with and look in the direction of Reiki and its source, then it will look at and

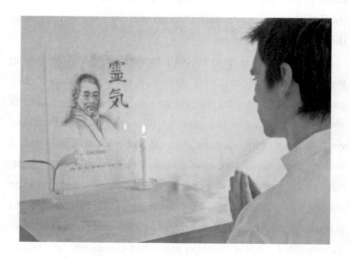

take note of you. If nothing happens, don't worry. Just make the connection to Reiki, open your heart, and ask for the unwanted energies of your patients to be removed from you. Believe in yourself and be patient with this method, as doubts may interfere with it. If you open your heart to the lineage, the bond will strengthen and the hearts of the Reiki lineage will fill with love.

Self-Treatments

The twenty-one-day cleanse using the twelve hand positions for self-treatment will bring to the surface your own mental, spiritual, emotional, and physical problems and allow the Reiki to work through your channels, energy field, and body. You may experience all manner of good and bad symptoms during a self-treatment. Both good and bad experiences give off emissions of light in your consciousness, but it is the level of light that gives definition.

The darkness that is released allows the light to flow through you more easily, and eventually it reveals the golden light beneath. When personal traumas are revealed and released during and after a treatment, don't consider them bad; instead, embrace them as precious moments that allow you to gain light, knowledge, insight, and experience along the spiritual path to healing and truth. These experiences are certainly no reason to give up on the practice.

Giving Reiki Treatments

Another interesting point about Reiki is that you do not lose anything by giving healing, because while you heal others, you also receive healing. Your heart opens to the divine, and much compassion and love flow through both you and your patient.

Healing with Reiki is a win-win process. Even if the client's ailment is not cured, both souls grow through that light. Reiki takes you beyond the healing of the body to the much higher plane of healing the soul. When the body dies, the soul retains the pains and impressions from its life on earth, and these elements are taken to the next birth to be played out in the soul's next life. It is this soul pain that is addressed through Reiki and that ultimately takes the individual to the "universal," so he or she may transcend the body and this world, but still be in it.

Meditations

The meditations and special breathing methods outlined in this book will bring you to a state of self-realization. With prolonged, disciplined, and gentle practice of Reiki methods, gradual layers of the personality or ego melt away. Then you may start to live life according to the soul that dwells in your body, so you may walk upon the earth, experience your desires, and fulfill your *dharma* (the karmic benefit you receive from doing good).

You may realize spiritual truths when going about your normal daily life, such as taking care of your children, doing your work, and spending time with your loved ones. These are all moments that give you the perfect opportunity to practice spiritual awakening by being fully present and aware of every action, thought, and emotion.

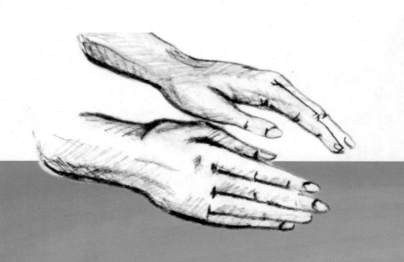

The Second Degree of Reiki: Okuden

11

The second-degree of Reiki is known as *okuden*, which means "inner teachings." In Japan, instruction for this level is usually broken into two parts, *kenki* (first) and *kouki* (second), and these two parts are taught over many years. However, in the West, the second degree is taught over two days during a ten- to twelve-hour teaching period.

I consider the inner teachings to be an introduction to the science of Reiki. At this level, you are given tools and methods that help you to understand and heal problems from your past, such as those having to do with emotions, mental habits, and cravings. You also learn a method of sending beneficial energy to your future. You are taught methods that help you to purify your soul, so that you can become one with the energies of the earth and Heaven, and truly experience a state of oneness.

Reiki Symbols: Shirushi Hô

Methods such as *shirushi hô* (the symbol method) allow you to access specific qualities and energies by focusing on a particular Sanskrit symbol or kanji character. Drawing the symbol correctly releases its energy, and its vitality is reinforced when you repeat its name a specific number of times. This allows you to draw on greater quantities of spiritual energy.

This book will not reveal the sacred Reiki symbols, which can only be received from a Master during training. However, one way to use the symbols method is to focus on the kanji symbols for Reiki itself. The symbol is broken into two parts, with the top part representing *rei*, which means "spiritual" or "soul," and the bottom part representing *ki*, which means "energy" and which consists of the vital forces of the earth and universe. This is how the symbols for "Reiki" would have been drawn around the time of Usui, although most of today's students will be used to the more modern form.

Rei = Spiritual

The Reiki symbols can be used as a focal point for meditation, because this process draws upon the vast ocean of Reiki. Concentrating on the symbol and repeating a mantra will channel a higher divine energy, and this will take you into higher states of consciousness. It can take no more than one dip into the vast spiritual ocean to achieve self-realization, and this insight is available to all who seek it.

Ki = Energy

At this point, you can choose to focus your attention on somebody who needs healing. Just maintain your awareness of that person and let the energy flow as it needs to, letting the Reiki move through you. You will be able to direct where the Reiki should flow, but bear in mind that to some extent, the Reiki consciousness will take charge. It will do what it needs for the person upon whom you are focusing. Symbols can be used as a healing tool for you and for others. They are the bridges of light that take the individual consciousness to the universal.

Reiki Mantras: Jumon and Kotodama

You will work with *jumon* (mantras) and *kotodama* (word spirit). These are sacred words that create and awaken energy channels within you. They contain certain energies, higher spiritual states, and spiritual truths. Through the process of opening your heart and repeating the mantras, the veil and illusions of this world will be gradually lifted, leading you to progressively higher states of clarity and spiritual truth. The mantras are like a rope that leads you out of the dark forest and back home to the true self, to happiness, love, and spiritual knowledge. With each repetition of a chosen mantra, you pull yourself along this rope, not exactly knowing where you are going, although you feel compelled to go there. Don't become too complacent. Maintain an open heart, keep your focus and faith, and don't forget your aim while repeating your mantra.

Meditation and Breathing Exercises

Methods of meditation and breathing exercises that were taught at the first level of Reiki are expanded at the second level; other aspects are added, creating a method called *hatsurei hô*. This method is a very powerful exercise that allows you to become more sensitive to Reiki. It opens the energy points in the heart and hands to a greater extent than before, producing a balance of mind, body, and emotions. It purifies and empowers the soul and creates a purposeful state of mind.

Distant Healing

Distant healing is useful for helping someone who can't come to you in person, and for sending energy to heal the traumas of your past. There are various ways of doing this. At the second level of Reiki, you would use the distant healing symbol. This symbol acts as a bridge between time and space, and it links the healer with the person receiving the healing. This is an advanced method that some second degree students learn, but I will show you a simpler method for giving distant healing.

A Simple Distant-Healing Method

1. Intend from your heart and soul your wish to connect to the lineage of Reiki, to Mikao Usui, to Reiki guides, to the Buddha, and to the source of Reiki. When you do this, the energy of the lineage protects and assists the healer and the healed with the highest intentions in mind for both.

2. Look at a photo of the person to whom you wish to send healing.

3. With your palms facing the photo, intend and project the energy into the photo, knowing in your heart that the energy is flowing to the person in mind for the highest good.

4. When you have finished, intend that Reiki is ending.

5. Mentally thank all those who assisted with this healing, for example, Reiki guides or spiritual beings.

It can be useful to become proficient in giving distant Reiki to family and friends first of all. Give your family member or friend distant Reiki while he or she lies on a sofa or a bed in another room. If this person doesn't live with you, make an arrangement over the phone so that you have a definite start and finish time, and ask this person to lie down so he or she will be relaxed during the distant Reiki treatment. You may even focus on particular spots on your friend's body while doing this. Be creative with this method and see what evolves.

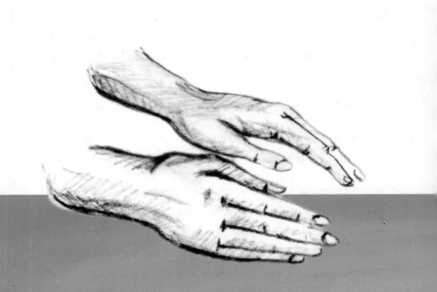

The Third Degree of Reiki: Shinpiden

12

The third degree is known as *shinpiden*, which in Japanese means "mystery teachings." In days gone by, students would have been given higher and deeper *reiju* empowerments to awaken and reinforce their connection to the Reiki source. Students were taught a fourth Reiki symbol, which came to be known as the "master symbol."

This level also assumed that the student wished to become a teacher. In the West, this level was altered so that students could receive this particular level of energy for personal spiritual growth and for healing others without becoming Reiki teachers.

Master Teacher: Shihan

The master teacher level is known as *shihan*, which means "teacher." This is as high as one can go in Reiki today, although there are Reiki specialists who think there is more to be revealed to us in the future.

At this level, you learn how to open your students' channels to Reiki, and you will be able to answer their questions and deal with their reactions in a controlled, relaxed, and safe environment. The master teacher level is about "becoming" the energy and about living it and letting it flow and direct you in your life on earth. It is a level of gradual surrender and melting of the ego.

Unfortunately in the West, just having the words "Reiki master" attached to one's name seems to be one of the biggest desires and a true reinforcement of many egos. The word "mastery" when applied to Reiki refers to the ongoing study and practice. Reaching this level in Reiki and receiving the title "master" is not an end result in itself, but just the beginning of a deeper journey. Real mastery is one of inner surrender and realization of the truth, rather than developing an overinflated opinion of oneself based on a fancy title.

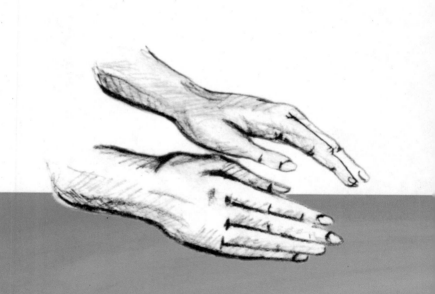

Reiki Methods

13

Reiki methods include meditation and breathing exercises, which are used to bring a shift in detachment, intuition, spiritual awakening, constant awareness, and spiritual truth. Following is an outline of some methods that are taught throughout all the levels of Reiki, and that are practiced for spiritual awakening and healing. I have explained some methods in enough detail for you to practice, but others are too complex for a book of this kind, so I have provided just enough information to give you a sense of them.

Reiji hô means "indication of the spirit." It is a way of praying and asking for Reiki to guide you through the day, during treatments, and in your practice. This connects Reiki energy to your heart and allows you to pass the Reiki through your hands and spiritual (third) eye.

Gasshô means "two hands coming together at the heart." This is also called the prayer posture in many Reiki traditions. This posture generates Reiki, and it allows you to detach from your mind. It strengthens intuition and balances the positive and negative poles in your body, creating a peaceful mind and unity of being.

Jôshin kokyû hû is a breathing exercise; the name means "breath spirit method" or "breathing exercise to purify the spirit." This exercise generates a large amount of Reiki within and outside the body. It cleanses and purifies the body, emotions, mind, and energy field, thus expanding your consciousness.

Hara mokunen is a method of focusing on the lower abdomen with the mind. *"Hara"* is an area or energetic center, and *"mokunen"* means "spirit focus and intent." This method builds great quantities of Reiki and brings balance and peace.

Kenyoku hô means "dry bathing" and is a way of purifying the soul and detaching from thoughts and emotions.

Kotodama means "word spirit" and is a word that contains specific energetic and divine vibrations. One chants it repetitively with feeling and devotion, using a specific breathing pattern. It will open you to Reiki and specific spiritual qualities.

Shirushi hô is a method of using ancient mystical symbols to produce certain spiritual and energetic qualities that you wish to develop within yourself.

Hatsurei hô means "generate spirit method." This enables you to generate a large amount of Reiki in and around the body. It opens specific energy channels, cultivates your heart and mind, and expands your consciousness.

Makoto no kokyu means "breath of truth." It is a self-healing method utilizing *kiko* exercises, breathing, meditation, *kotodama*, and *mudras* (hand gestures). This method is practiced to build huge amounts of "golden *ki*" in and around the body, focusing and defining the lower *hara* in the abdomen.

Reiju means "spiritual blessing or gift." A *reiju* empowerment is used to initiate and empower you with Reiki, to awaken you spiritually and open your energy channels. It can bring profound states of peace and bliss. Karma may be released and experienced during and after the empowerment, as this is part of a purification process. *Reiju* can be invoked and experienced during meditation to help reinforce your practice.

Practicing the Reiki Methods

The following methods will give you a feel for the study of Reiki and start you off on your spiritual path.

When practicing any of these methods, you access an elevated spiritual energy, which brings lower, denser energies to the surface. You may feel angry, resentful, unhappy, or off kilter, or you may suddenly find yourself remembering past hurts. The *gasshô* method helps you to detach from these reactions. Just experience the feelings without judging or reacting. For example, if you encounter sadness, don't dwell on it or analyze it. Accept the sadness; know that it will pass and that your true nature is blissful and not attached to the sadness, or to any other stray emotion that arises at this time. Don't stop meditating or studying Reiki, because you will soon be able to handle these feelings as your inner strength increases.

If you stop the practice now, you will always associate Reiki with sadness, depression, and pain, and this would be a shame. Work through this phase, and most of all, be patient and kind to yourself and to your clients.

I have put these methods in an order of practice, as the power grows as you progress. This order provides you with a safe method of progressing.

Meditation Posture

In Japan these methods are used while the practitioner is sitting on the knees in the *seiza* (correct sitting) posture. You can choose to sit in the lotus posture instead, with your legs crossed and with your feet placed on each thigh with your soles facing upward. If you are stiff and unused to exercise, sit upright on the edge of a chair with your back straight and without touching the chair back, or sit in a relaxed cross-legged posture.

1. Kneel in *seiza* posture, with your feet tucked under you, leaving about two hands' width between your knees. Your

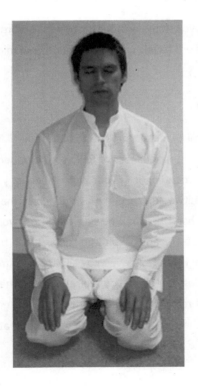

weight should be evenly distributed on your buttocks, and not too far back or forward on your legs.

2. Place your hands palm down on your thighs.

3. Your spine should be straight, as if floating via a golden thread coming from above your head, through your crown, and down the center of your body, stopping at the *hara* (lower abdomen), where the *tanden* (energy point) is located.

4. Lower your chin slightly and fix your eyes on the floor a few feet ahead of you. Your eyes should be relaxed and partially closed.

5. Focus your mind on your nostrils as you breathe in and out, as this will have a calming effect on your mind.

Reiji Hô

The term *reiji hô* means "indication of the spirit." It is a method of bringing the consciousness of Reiki to the upper *tanden* (energy point) and grounding it in your heart, opening you up to higher spiritual intuitive guidance. It was the hub of the system of Usui *teate* (Usui hand healing), healing based on working intuitively on a person by means of spirit guidance. It can be used to guide you in many ways, from everyday situations to meditation, healing and taking you along your spiritual path. There are different methods of *reiji hô*; the method described here is an extended version of the traditional methods of focusing at just the upper *tanden* or the middle *tanden*.

1. This method can be practiced standing, seated in the *seiza* posture, or in any other comfortable position.

2. Bring your two hands, palms together, to your heart in the prayer position (*gasshô*). Mentally say, "*Reiji hô* is starting now" or "Reiki is starting now."·

3. Mentally ask the Reiki to enter your heart, and then feel the energy and connection that allow Reiki to flow from your hands and heart. Say, "I open my heart and soul to Reiki. Please fill me with love, light, compassion, and enlightened activity."

4. Keep your hands in the prayer position, but move them up to your throat so that you can feel the flow of energy and connection of Reiki in your hands and throat. Mentally say, "Please fill my speech with the Reiki light, and guide me with compassionate, loving, and enlightened speech."

5. With your hands still in the prayer position, take them up to your spiritual eye, located between your eyebrows. Feel the flow of energy and the connection between your hands and your spiritual eye. Mentally say, "Please fill my spiritual eye with Reiki and guide me on my spiritual path upon the earth."

    Here are four examples of intentions that you can make with your hands at the heart or spiritual eye.

I open my heart and soul to Reiki.
Please guide me on my spiritual path.

Reiki, please fill my heart and soul and
guide me with this healing.

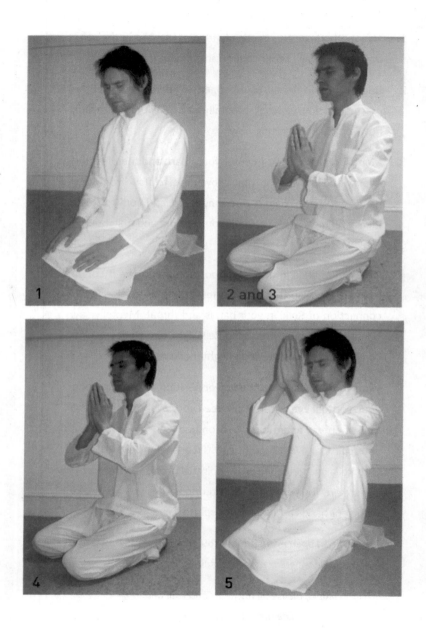

> *Reiki, fill my heart and soul and guide me*
> *upon the earth in peace and love.*

> *Reiki, fill my heart and soul and guide me so I can*
> *fulfill my life purpose on the earth.*

6. With your hands still in the prayer position, move them gently back down in front of your heart and mentally say, "*Reiji hô* is ending now."

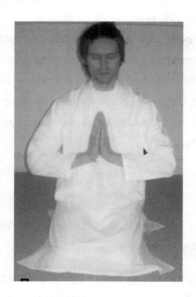

Gasshô

The *gasshô* method is introduced during the first degree of Reiki; it means "two hands coming together at the heart." It is used in conjunction with many other exercises, including the *reiju* empowerment, which opens, empowers, and reinforces your connection to Reiki. It is a very important meditation, which uses the ancient hand gesture that relates to Kannon, which means "the Compassionate Buddha," and Dai-Seishi Bosatsu, which means "the Buddha of Wisdom."

This hand position brings certain states of consciousness and qualities represented by Buddha. It opens and balances many energy channels in and around the body. In conjunction with the hand posture, the mind is used to focus on the pulse in the fingers. This allows the Reiki to accumulate in and around you while your mind is focused.

1. Kneel with your feet tucked under you in *seiza* or in any other comfortable position.

2. You may intend that Reiki is starting or flowing. Mentally affirm this when you are sitting comfortably.

3. Put your hands together in the prayer posture, and place them at the center of your chest (sternum), where the middle *tanden* is located.

4. Become aware of the gentle pulse at your two middle fingertips.

5.   Let all your thoughts come and go, so that you become an observer and detach yourself from your thoughts.

6.   Don't judge any of your thoughts; just watch them pass by, and maintain your focus upon the pulse in your middle fingers.

7.   If your mind wanders, gently bring your awareness back to focus on the pulse in your middle fingers.

8.   Practice this method for ten to fifteen minutes.

Sensations and Experiences

During this meditation, you may feel fatigue in your arms because they are unused to the posture, but this will subside with time. You will also notice the amount of "chatter" your mind creates; this method is just what is needed to stop that. Your hands may become hot and they may tingle, and there will be a buildup of heat inside your body that may come in waves or hot flushes. While you focus on the pulse in your fingertips, you may notice your whole body pulsing in synchronization. Your intuition will become heightened over time.

This exercise makes you feel calm and balanced. If you encounter heat and emotions afterward, they will eventually subside when your energy channels become unblocked. This is a temporary emotional upheaval on the road to balance. You may encounter detachment and moments of stillness and deep peace.

Jôshin Kokyû Hô

The name of this method means "breath spirit method." It is used to bring spiritual energy down into the body via the crown of the head, so that it can flow throughout and beyond the body in all directions. The aim is to spiritualize and purify the body, the energy field, and the soul. This method will build great amounts of spiritual energy in and around the body and will expand your consciousness. It creates peace of mind and acts as an internal space clearer, leaving you in a state of emptiness so that you can see and acknowledge the true spirit.

1. Kneel with your feet tucked under you or in any other comfortable position, keeping your back straight.

2. Rest your hands, palms facing up, on your thighs.

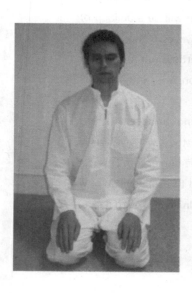 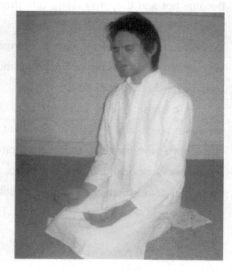

3. Silently intend that Reiki is starting.

4. Focus your mind above the crown of your head.

5. Breathe naturally through your nose.

6. When you inhale, visualize a golden stream of energy flooding into your crown and filling your body.

7. Pause for a couple of seconds so that you can visualize and feel the light energy flooding your body.

8. When you exhale, visualize and feel the light rays expand through and beyond your body in all directions as far as your imagination will take you (for instance, into your street, into space, into the universe, and so on).

9. During this exhalation and visualization, you may feel all your tensions being washed away. Relax as you exhale.

10. Repeat this method at least sixteen times.

11. Finish by silently intending that Reiki is ending now.

This method will induce a state of inner space and peace. Your skin will feel refreshed, soft, and smooth, as it is coated with a layer of spiritual energy. A great amount of internal heat is accumulated while practicing this method, yet afterward your body may feel cold. This is because the sitting posture, breathing, and visualization build and lock Reiki into the body.

Once the method is complete and you start to move around again, the energy moves through and around the body, making you feel cool. You will really feel clean internally and externally as the soul is washed with spiritual energy.

Hara Breathing

Focusing and breathing into the lower *hara* (abdomen) allows you to become balanced and detached from any unbalancing emotions and situations. If excess energy causes mental, physical, or emotional discomfort, focus on this area and the energy will draw back into its "storehouse," where it can't cause mischief. This area allows great quantities of energy to be stored; it is also the crossroads where many energy channels meet. Reiki can be stored at this point, so that a gradual buildup will rise through the spine to the brain, passing through the lower, middle, and upper energy spots in the process. This leads to moments of spiritual awakening. Your hands placed at this point will bring Reiki through your palms into your *hara*.

1. Kneel with your feet tucked under you in *seiza* posture or any of the other recommended positions.

2. Gently focus your eyes while they are half-closed and look down to the floor about three feet (a little less than a meter) in front of you. Alternatively, you may close your eyes.

3. Mentally say, "Reiki is starting now."

4. Focus your attention on the breath entering and leaving your nostrils for a few minutes to calm your mind.

5. Place your right palm on the lower *hara* and place your left hand on top of your right.

6. Focus your mind at the point internally where your hands are placed on your lower *hara*.

7. As you breathe naturally through your nose, maintain your focus at the lower *hara*, and become aware of the gentle motion of your abdomen expanding with the inhalations and contracting with the exhalations.

8. Practice this method for ten to fifteen minutes.

Conclusion

Through this book, I have tried to provide a simple explanation of a spiritual healing and meditation system whose popularity is still increasing. It emerged from the uncluttered purity of Japanese mysticism. Reiki has been adapted by the various New Age movements and diluted by a variety of beliefs, but now the approach to this system has come full circle and many people are returning to its Japanese roots. This book aims to give you the meditating and healing system that draws directly from the Japanese teachings.

This book will give you a safe foundation and will introduce you to most of the teachings at the first degree, called *shoden*. The Reiki meditations and breathing exercises should help you to center your mind, build up and expand the Reiki, and—a very important benefit—allow you to detach from the ego and distinguish your spiritual self. Most important, Reiki is for everybody, regardless of experience, race, faith, or status. Everyone who embraces this practice will develop peace, love, and spiritual truth, which flow naturally from the consciousness of Reiki. Ten years of Reiki practice and experience have shown me many times that Reiki is a complementary system that blends well with other healing arts and spiritual systems.

Reiki seems to be able to alleviate the suffering that so many people experience in their lives, and it leads them to a place that I call "true happiness." This is a space in the heart that can be found at the interface of happiness and sadness, and which is a lasting, unconditional state of consciousness. May you find this true happiness through the prolonged practice of the Reiki methods in this book, and by offering yourself to the world as a tool for healing and inspiration.

Other Titles in the *Plain & Simple* Series

Hampton Roads Publishing Company

. . . *for the evolving human spirit*

Hampton Roads Publishing Company publishes books on
a variety of subjects, including spirituality, health,
and other related topics.

For a copy of our latest catalog, call (978) 465-0504 or visit our
distributor's website at *www.redwheelweiser.com*. You can also
sign up for our newsletter and special offers by going to
www.redwheelweiser.com/newsletter

3 1333 04607 4611